The Inner Secrets

Perfect Eyesight

The Art of Improving Vision Naturally

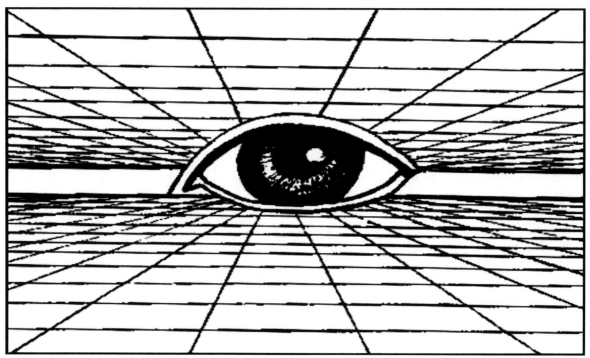

A Complete Course in Eyesight Healing

Robert A. Zuraw and Robert T. Lewanski, aka: R.T. Lewis
A health and eyesight healing book from

Taoist Publishers ☯ Troy, Michigan 48083

INFORMATION DISCLAIMER

This book does not represent, in any way, orthodox medical opinion. The findings herein presented are all natural methods as passed down from the wisest and most knowledgeable men and women throughout history. The material in this book is presented as educational information, and no claim is made as to what the methods cited herein may do for an individual in any given case. You should not use this information to diagnose or treat any health or eye problems or illnesses without consulting your holistic health care provider or holistic medical doctor. Please consult a competent holistic physician with any questions or concerns you might have regarding your eyes or any health conditions you may have. The information on this book is not intended as a substitute for the advice of a physician, eye specialist, or holistic health care provider. This information is not intended as a substitute for the reader's independent judgment and personal responsibility. Health issues are far too important to delegate to anyone else. It is highly recommended you research and seek information and counsel from as wide a variety of sources as possible, so you can make well informed educated decisions about your health, as in the end YOU make the decisions. The authors and publishers assume no obligation or liability as to how any one may use or misuse this information. Those with eye injuries, eye diseases, and/or degenerative eye conditions consult with a professional eye specialist or physician. The Dietary Supplement Health and Education Act (DSHEA) of 1994 requires us to state: "These statements have not been evaluated by the Food and Drug Administration. These products are not intended to diagnose, treat, cure, or prevent any disease."

ACKNOWLEDGMENTS

We would like to thank first of all, Jason Schofield for his untiring efforts to get this computer beast up and running; for his help in computer scanning images. Thanks to Tim Trikes for his back cover work. And to Stef Chura for her help with uploading dreamstime.com front cover picture. To Joe Alexander for interior art work. We also owe a debt of gratitude to all the great teachers of natural eye training throughout history who have given us hope and insight into holistic health and vision training practices. And to all the wise holistic health doctors and teachers who, over the years, helped us formulate the health, diet, herb, body typing and chi kung principles that went into this eye course. A special thanks to our parents who brought us here for this purpose, and who gave us the freedom to grow and learn on our own. We also acknowledge and dedicate this book to all those sovereign, free thinking individuals throughout the world who are seeking higher wisdom and the freedom to express their creativity in natural and spiritual ways. And above all, we are grateful and thankful for the Creative Force of Heaven and Earth who gave us this opportunity to discover, learn and teach these principles, so that others' may also benefit from them. Thanks to our good friends and students who have supported us in our endeavors. It is with much love and affection that we share our discoveries with you.

Library of Congress Catalog Card Number: 98-60555
1. Perfect Eyesight. 2. Health. 3. Oriental/Ayurveda Medicine.
4. Diet. 5. Herbs. 6. Exercise 7. Vision. 8. Eyes. I. Title
First Edition 1999. Second Edition 2001. Third Edition 2007. Fifth Edition 2011.
Website: www.healthforcecenter.com

Illustrations and inside front cover design by Joseph Alexander
New front and back cover layout work by Tim Trikes
Initial computer setup and scanning by Jason Schofield
A special acknowledgment and thanks to Tim Trikes, who graphically set up the back book cover. His company does graphic design, manufactures and installs all types of signs and offers design orientated solutions. Trikes Sign Company 33200 W. Nine Mile Rd., Farmington, MI (48336)
248-476-0033

No part of this book may be reproduced, stored in a retrieval system, or transmitted
by any means without the written permission of the author.
First published by Taoist Publishers
Printed in the United States of America
2011 Robert T. Lewanski© All rights reserved.

ISBN - 13: 9781456475680   ISBN - 10-1456475681

What This Book Can Do For You

You are about to embark on a sacred journey: a Vision Quest into the world of crystal clear eyesight, health rejuvenation and unlimited energy. It is a journey you have to take all by yourself! No one else can give you Perfect Eyesight, super-health or bursting energy. You and only *you* must acquire the knowledge, wisdom and understanding to apply these teachings to your life. Nothing in life is free. There is always a price to pay through effort or sweat equity. However, the rewards are satisfying; freedom from bother-some eye glasses or contacts; saving thousands of dollars over a lifetime of purchasing eyewear; **freedom from disease, crystal clear vision, and unlimited bounding health and energy.** Isn't this worth living for?

There are many books written on eyesight improvement and holistic health. However, awaiting you is a rare experience! Never before has a book been written encompassing the health-connection relationship between body, mind, eyes. Eastern cultures and religions **do not separate** the body, mind, and spirit. They see the person and the whole of existence as ONE. What effects one part, effects the whole. They have practiced and taught a holistic view of health and the universe for thousands of years. The word health means to be whole and complete in body, mind and spirit. This holistic view of life also includes the eyes, which they consider to be "the windows of the soul."

Here in this enlightening, inspiring and informative book you will discover long-lost formulas and secret eye-health teachings. These secrets have been taught by masters, holistic health practitioners, eye specialists and eye doctors throughout the ages.

For the first time in one book you will discover how the three main Ayurvedic body types—Air(Vata), Fire(Pitta) and Water(Kapha)—effect ones' health and eyesight. Your health and vision can zoom when you consume the correct foods for your individual constitutional body type.

Discovering and applying this information can make the difference between dim failing eyesight and health, and unlimited zestful and youthful vitality. Perfect eyesight can be retained far into advanced age. This is no idle boast. We challenge you to prove and test these teachings for yourself. Take nothing for granted. "Prove all things, hold fast to that which is true."

The excitement doesn't stop there! Further discover special **Chi Kung Energy Exercises and Do-In (Dao-Yin) Self-Massage Techniques.** These special techniques are designed to boost your internal energy, improve glandular function, enhance hormones, and circulate rich red oxygen-filled blood to your eyes and brain. You'll actually begin to think, feel and look young again! Again, no idle chatter! Perform these Secret Oriental Chi Kung Movements and feel your energy, eyesight, and spirit skyrocket! They are fun and easy to do. You'll also disc over how to stay grounded, centered and balanced; to remain strong and alert; develop your intuition, intelligence and physical strength. Plus, discover special herbs, tonics and foods to detoxify
your liver and cleanse your body, which helps to improve vision.

Life takes on a new meaning for you. You begin to spiral upward to a new awareness and a higher sense of self. Because of your newfound purpose in life--increased wisdom, understanding, knowledge, along with practice--your vision begins to improve. You begin to "see" things clearly, not only visually, but spiritually and intuitively.

You'll be introduced to proven principles, the personal application of which can literally transform your vision, if you persistently and consistently practice them. All of the eye, health and chi kung techniques have been tested and proven safe for both beginner and advanced student—young or old. You can progress as far as you wish to go in regaining or maintaining superb vision, health, beauty, strength and fitness.

Every day that you apply these powerful eye and health techniques, you will build and improve your life. So why not start today, right now, and decide that you too can benefit by these wonderful restorative methods--and discover for yourself what a dramatic transformation they
will bring into your life.

Then let others marvel at the results you have achieved. May you attain the Perfect Eyesight and super-health you are seeking! Turn the page to Chapter One and begin your vision and health improvement quest today!

Robert T. Lewanski,
President,Taoist Publishers
Troy, Michigan
July 30, 2011

FORWARD
Discover the Real Secrets of How You Can Attain Perfect Eyesight Without Glasses or Surgery!

Yes, he quit wearing eye-glasses and he attained 20-20 vision in both eyes. You too can stop wearing eye-glasses and regain normal vision. Wouldn't it be wonderful to no longer have to wear cumbersome eye glasses. And the best part of it is--that you will see better, than ever before, by following the real inner secrets of Perfect Eyesight,.

He was eager to tell his story--and why not for he had been wearing eye- glasses for years and had been told by eye doctors that he would always have to wear them. But, he followed the advice of Natural Eyesight Improvement Specialists and discovered the real truth about eyes.

Robert Zuraw discovered the method for strengthening the eyes and correcting eye troubles that is now acclaimed by many thousands who have tested it and found it of untold benefit.

Thousands of people go through life with the belief that they have to wear eye-glasses not knowing that Natural Eye Science now offers them normal vision through a simple system of natural eye correction, outlined in these pages.

Why suffer with unnecessary eye problems?

Truly a revelation. And what a sense of accomplishment and satisfaction. Think of it. After being a slave to eye-glasses for years--you can discard your glasses forever. Building up the strength of your eyes can be an enjoyable process—that doesn't take much time to perform. Only a few short months, in most cases, of self-treatment, in correct eye exercise techniques—eye supplements and natural habits, can improve your vision tremendously.

The world today is full of men and women who endure unnecessary suffering because of poor eyesight. They think that glasses will cure or eliminate the conditions responsible for eye troubles! But glasses are nothing more than eye crutches. The real help must come from other sources. In the case of the eyes, it is exercise, good health and diet habits, and corrective eye habits.

How one man went from "legal blindness" without glasses to 20-20 perfect vision

Over 40 years ago, Robert Zuraw had a most trying experience with his eyes--he was legally blind without glasses. Eye doctors gave him no hope of ever improving his vision or discarding his glasses. That was enough for him. He knew there had to be someone who could help him. He was not yet ready to throw in the towel. He was a fighter--a real street fighter in his youth. His determined will-power kicked-in. The idea of wearing glasses was intolerable, absolutely annoying. Always willing to back up his theories by experimenting upon himself, he immediately searched and eventually found Natural Eye Improvement Specialists, and started in upon a course of natural eye treatment that he fully believed would help him.

With the help of Natural Eye Trainers, plus books and eye courses from around the world, he entered upon a period of research and experiment covering 30 years. The results were so entirely satisfactory that he associated himself with two of the few really great natural eye specialists and his vision zoomed from 20-600 to 20-20, and to 30-10, better than 20-20. His vision improved, even at the 50 and 60 year old mark!

A startling revolutionary system of eye training

Upon their findings, and his incredible reversal of advanced myopia, has risen, like a Phoenix from the ashes, a remarkable new scientific system of eye training which quickly enables you to train the muscles of the eyes so that you too can make them work properly at all times, and without effort or strain. This new system has been discovered by Robert Zuraw, in collaboration with the latest scientific natural eyesight discoveries, worldwide, and the editing and research help of Robert T. Lewanski, aka: R.T. Lewis.

Now, you too can discover the real truth
about how the eyes really work!

If you already wear glasses, find out how you can discard them. If you do not wear glasses, but feel that your sight is failing, then find out how a few minutes each day assures you perfect sight without the use of glasses. If you are a parent, send at once for this method, and learn how to save your children from the scourge of poor eyesight-- how you can save them from the slavery of eye-glasses. Learn how thousands of other people regained normal vision.

Throw your glasses or contacts away, forever!
Eye glasses and contacts are only crutches anyway

Here is a man who writes: "By faithfully following the directions given in your "Perfect Eyesight" book, I have discarded glasses worn for years."

Another grateful reader of the "Perfect Eyesight" book writes: "I had been wearing glasses since I was eight years old and could not go a day without them. I am now twenty-four and with just a little effort in practicing the Eye Exercises each week for a period of two months, I have been able to stop wearing glasses entirely."

These inspiring results bring a message of hope to everyone who is troubled with weak eyes or poor sight. There is hardly any condition (except degenerative chronic eye disease) that is beyond the reach of Robert Zuraw's revolutionizing "Perfect Eyesight" method of eye training.

Table of Contents

Introduction, 1

Chapter One: The Miracle of Perfect Eyesight, 6
- The Truth About the Eyes, 6 - Eye Muscles Accommodation: The Mystery Unveiled, 7 - How Good is Your Peripheral Vision?, 7 - A Quick Lesson in Eye Anatom, 8 - Eye Retina's "Yellow Spot" Secret to Vision, 9 - Oriental Eye and Health Diagnosis, 9 - How the Eyes "See", 10 - Are Eye Glasses or Contacts Necessary?, 10 - How Long Does it Take to Achieve 20-20 Vision?, 11

Chapter Two: Daily Eye Strengthening Habits, 13
- Practice Distance Seeing, 13 - What Causes Weak Eye Muscles?, 14, - Look Up from Your Close Work, 14, - Avoid Close Work During and After Meals, 15 - Fourteen Eye Habits For Perfect Eyesight: Eye Habit number One: Do not read when tired or sick, 15 - Eye Habit Number Two: Do not read more than thirty minutes at a time, 17 - Eye Habit Number Three: The Invigorating Lemon Juice Eye Bath, 17 - Eye Habit Number Four: Healing Sun Part 1: Sunshine is Food for the Eyes, 18 – Healing Sun Part II: Secrets of Yoga Sun Gazing, 18 – Healing Sun Part III: Sunglasses Harmful? – Eye Habit Number Five: The Oriental 'Yang Eye' Candle Gazing Technique, 19 Eye Habit Number Six: The East Indian Yoga Nasal Massage Technique, 20 – Eye Habit Number Seven: Chinese Taoist Kidney, Stomach and Liver Massage, 20 – Eye Habit Number Eight: Acupressure Eye Massage and Eye Palming Techniques, 21 – Eye Habit Number Nine: Neck Loosening Exercises, 21- Eye Habit Number Ten: Taoist Dao-Yin Eye Massage Techniques, 22 – Eye Massage Technique A: Chinese Scalp Rubbing Eye Technique, 22 – Eye Massage Technique B: Palm Eye Massage Technique, 22 – Eye Massage Technique C: Stroking Eyebrows Technique, 23 – Eye Massage Technique D: Ironing the Face Technique, 23 – Eye Habit Number Eleven: Squeeze Eyes Tightly and Open Eyes Widely, 23 – Eye Habit Number Twelve: Naturopathic Eye Massage Technique, 23 – Eye Habit Number Thirteen: Tracking or Edging: The Secret to Crystal Sharp Vision, 24 – Eye Habit Number Fourteen: Head Lift Technique for Eye and Ear Problems, 25

Chapter Three: Perfect Eyesight Exercise Techniques, 26
– Eye Exercise Protocol, 27 – "Lazy Eight" Neck Loosing Exercise (Pre-Eye Exercise Warm-up Technique), 27 – Eye Exercise One: Egyptian Black Dot Technique – Part I (Eye Muscle Exercise), 28 – Egyptian Black Dot Technique – Part II, 28 – Eye Exercise Two: Egyptian Letter Gazing Technique – Part I (Eye Muscle Exercise for Close and Distant Vision), 29 – Advanced Egyptian Letter Gazing Technique – Part II, 30 – Eye Exercise Three: Yoga Accommodative Eye Exercise (To Improve Close and Distant Vision), 31 – Eye Exercise Four: Yoga Accommodative Eye Exercise (To Improve Distant Vision), 32 – Eye Exercise Five: Tai Chi Rocker Eye Technique—An Amazing Discovery (To Improve Close and Distant Vision), 32 – Chart 1: Snellen Eye Chart Test Card, 34 – Points to Remember While Performing the Tai Chi Rocker Technique, 35 – Eye Exercise Six: Close Vision Strengthening Exercises: Close Vision Technique A: (Accommodative "Whipping Eye Technique"), 35 – Close Vision Technique B: "Tromboning", 36 – Close Vision: Chart 2: Principles of Eye Training Chart, 38 – Eye Exercise Seven: Stretch Your Vision: Distant Vision Strengthening Exercise (To Improve Nearsightedness—Myopia), 39 – Eye Exercise Seven: Test Card Eye Exercise (To Improve Close and Distant Vision), 41 – Distant Vision Exercise, 42 – Eye Exercise Eight: Tibetan Peripheral Vision Technique, 42 – Eye Exercise Nine: Dr. Bates' and Yoga Eye Palming Techniques, 44 – Palming Soothes and Rests the Eyes, 44 – "Let Go" Mentally While Palming, 44 – How to Perform the Yoga Fetal Palming Technique, 45 – Heal Liver and Eyes with the Color of Green, 46 – The Sit Down Palming Technique, 46 – The Secret 'Black Globe' Palming Technique, 46 – The Key to Seeing Perfect Blackness, 47 – The Amazing Master Formulas Behind "Perfect Eyesight", 47 – The Three Master Formulas to Perfect Eyesight: Master Eye Formula Number One: Relax the Eye Muscles, 47 – Master Eye Formula Number Two: Relax the Brain and Mind, 48 – Master Eye Formula Number Three: Reduce Mental Strain and Strengthen Eye Muscles, 48 – What is Progressive Eye Training?, 48 – Eyesight Training Exercise Schedule: Weekly Eye Training Program, 49 – Daily Eye Training Program, 49

Chapter Four: Internal Chi Kung Energy Exercises For Vision Improvement,
50 – How to Build a Strong Healthy Constitution, 50 - Internal Exercise Number One: Kidney and Lower Back Strengthening Movement, 50 – Internal Exercise Number Two: Spine Straightening Movement, 51 – Internal Exercise Number Three: Reaching for Heaven, 51 – Internal Exercise Number Four: Tibetan Rejuvenation Rite, 52 – Internal Exercise Number Five: Sufi Bear Walk (Egyptian), 52 – Internal Exercise Number Six: Jade Hop, 53 – Internal Exercise Number Seven: Centering Movement, 53

Chapter Five: Special Oriental Dao-Yin: Self-Healing Massage for Healthy Eyesight,
55 – Vision Health and Healing Secrets, 55 – Daily Oriental Dao-Yin Self-Healing Massage Routine, 56 – Dao-Yin (Self-Massage) Helps Clear Energy Blockages for Eye and Brain Healing, 57 – Healing Hara-Belly Massage, 57 – The Three Power Centers, 57 – The Heart and the Belly, 58 – Hara Massage for Unlimited Energy, 58 – Foot Slapping to Invigorate the Kidneys and Nourish the Eyes and Liver: Traditional Chinese Medical Chi Kung Dao-Yin Technique to Improve Mental Health, Energy and Vision, 59 – Positive Benefits of Foot Slapping or Tapping, 59 – A Personal Experience of Foot Slapping, 60 – Overcoming Depression and Emotional Problems with Foot Slapping, 60 – The Hara, Brain Activity and Visual Clarity, 60 – Balancing Upper and Lower Body Centers, 61 – How to Perform the Foot Slapping Dao-Yin Technique to Strengthen the Kidneys and Adjust your Energy Levels, 61 – Point of Attention, 62 – Foot Slapping Balances Water and Fire in the Body, 62

Chapter Six: Nutritional Secrets for Visual Clarity,
63 – Healing Your Eyesight and Body with Whole Foods, 63 – "Physician, Heal Thyself", 64 – Discover the Inner Secrets of Health, Nutrition and Unlimited Energy: The Five Health-Nutrition Keys to Perfect Eyesight: Health Key Number One—Eat only when hungry and drink liquids only when thirsty, 64 – Health Key Number Two—Chew our Food Well—Your Key to Good Eyesight and Health, 66 – Health Key Number Three—Eat Mostly Whole Natural Foods in Season and in Your Climate, 67 – Health Key Number Four—Super-Nutrient-Rich Foods for Perfect Eyesight, 68 – Herbs to Heal and Protect the Liver and Vision, 68 – Foods That Heal, Cleanse and Strengthen the Liver and Eyes, 69 – Health Key Number Four—Toxic Foods That Cause Ill Health and Vision Problems, 69 – Sugar Blues, Depression andMyopia (Nearsightedness), 70 – Excess Salt and Weak Vision, 71 – White Flour and Poor Vision, 71 – Fats and Oils in the Blood, 71 – GMO Non-Organic Soybean Products CAN Cause Toxic Blood and Weak Vision, 72 – Oils, Vision Defects, Balding and Immune System Deficiencies, 73 – Vegetarians Beware of GMO Foods and Isolated Soy Products, 73 – The Ill-Effects of Rapeseed(Canola Oil) and Soy Oil on Liver, Blood, Eyes and Health, by John Thomas, Author of "Young Again", 74 – Non-Organic, Non-Fermented Soy Isolates Cause of Deranged Digestion, 75 – Genetically Modified Soy Protein is Not a Growth Protein, 75 – Important Health Note on Oils, Caution!, 75 – Use Healthy Oils Moderately for Good Vision and Health—The Best Oils: Olive, Sesame, Sunflower, Coconut, Flax, Grapeseed, 76

Chapter Seven: A Complete Protocol and Analysis of Nutritional Body Types for Optimum Health and Perfect Eyesight,
77 – Ayurvedic Nutritional Body Typing Health System Protocol 77 – A Complete Anakysis and Protocol for (Kapha) Water Body Type—(Watery, Crusty, Expanded Eyes), 78 – Characteristics of a Kapha-Water Body Type, 78 – Kapha-Water Body Types Need Less Water, Not More, 79 – The Potato Juice Eye Bath for Watery Eyes, 79 – Kapha-Water Body Type Foods—Avoid These Foods if You Have Watery Eyes, 80 – Foods That Reduce Water and Mucus for the Water Body Type, 80 – Complete Dietary Requirements: Foods, Herbs, Vitamins, Minerals and Supplements for Kapha-Water Type, 81 – Special Therapies to Reduce Kapha-Water Body Type, 83 – How Much Water Do You Really Need?, 83 – A Complete Analysis and Protocol for Vata-Air Body Type—(Dry,Twitching, Itchy and Contracted Eyes), 84 – Vata-Air Body Type—Avoid These Food if You Have Dry Eyes, 84 – Warming, Moisturizing, Grouding Foods to Balance the Vata-Air Body Type, 85 – Complete Dietary Requirements: Foods, Herbs, Vitamins, Minerals and Supplements for Vata-Air Body Type, 86 – Special Therapies to Increase Moisture and Warmth in Vata-Air Body Types, 87 – A Complete Analysis and Protocol for Pitta-Fire Body Type—(Hot, Stinging, Red Inflamed eyes or Conjunctivitis), 87 – Pitta-Fire Body Type Foods—Avoid These Foods if You Have Inflamed Red, Stinging Eyes, 88 – Foods to Cool and Balance the Pitta-Fire Body Type, 88 – Complete Dietary Requirements: Foods, Herbs, Vitamins, Minerals and

Supplements for Pitta-Fire Body Type, 89 – Special Therapies to Reduce Heat and Inflammation in Pitta-Fire BodyTypes, 90 – (See APPENDIX D for Nutritional Body Typing over the Phone and email Consultations or Information), 91 - The Eye – Xerciser, 92

Chapter Eight: Three Extraordinary "Ten Minute" Eye Improvement Techniques, 93

– Sunning, Palming and the Long Swing, 93 – Eye Technique Number One—The "Sunning Technique, 94 – Eye Technique Number Two—The "Palming" Technique, 95 – Eye Technique Number Three—The "Long Swing" Technique, 95 – The "Black Period" Eye-Gazing Technique—For Sharpening Close and Distant Vision, 97 -

Chapter Nine: Do You Really Want Perfect Eyesight?, 99

– Short and Medium Eye Routine for Those with Busy Schedules, 100 – The Short Eye Exercise Routine—Fifteen minutes, three times a week, 100 – The Medium Eye Exercise Routine—Forty minutes, two times a week, 100 – Woman Does Eye Routine Only Once a Week and Improves Her Vision Dramatically!, 100 – Lady Throws Glasses Away After Only One Eyesight Training Session, 101 – Perform the Eye Routines with Fun, Joy and Relaxation, 101 – Avoid 'Squinting' as Much as Possible, 101 – Arching the Eyebrows, 101 – Sinus Problems, Dry or Watery Eyes, 102 – Too Much Close Work Weakens Distant Vision, 102 – A Stressful Life and its Effect Upon Vision, 102 – Eye Exercises and Moderation: How Much is Enough?, 103 – Think on the Things You Want, 103 – How to Overcome Discouragement, 104 – The Magic Formula for Success, 104 – The Empty Mind Technique, 105 – Sufi Mind-Eye Breathing Technique, 105 – The Tranquil Meditation Technique, 106

Chapter Ten: Vision Wisdom from Holistic Health and Natural Eye Specialists, 108

– Eyes Reflect the Health of the Body, 108 – Clean Out Your Bloodstream and Improve Your Vision, 109 – Get Fitted for Weaker Lenses, 109 – The Day Dreamer, 109 – Vision is Your Most Precious Possession, 109 – Comb Your Hair and Improve Your Eyesight, 110 – Distant Vision Exercise: See Like a Telescope With Your Naked Eye, 110 – Strengthen Your Stomach and Improve Your Vision, 110 – How to Prevent Eye Strain and Defective Eyes With the "Alternate Gaze Technique", 110 – Look Up FromYour Close Work, 111 – Discover Dr. Peppard's Secret to Prevent "Nearsightedness", 111 – Strengthen Your Eye Muscles for Perfect Eyesight, 112 – The "Exhaling Bull" Technique for Eye Power and Rejuvenation, 112 – To "Blink" or Not to "Blink" that is the Question!, 113 – Eye-Blinking Linked to Inner Health, Energy and Personal Magnetism, 113 – Diet and Dao-Yin: Health Diagnosis Through the Eyes, 114 – Heed the Warning: Unfermented GMO Soybeans, Soy Oil, Soy Milk, Tofu Linked to Thyroid Problems, Protruding Eyes, Liver Disease and Weak Immunity, 115 – Ancient Zen-Taoist Technique to Reduce Swollen Eyes, 115 – The "Eye-Power-Gaze" Technique, 116 – The Secret of the "Steady Eye", 116 – A Naturopathic Cure for Weak Eyesight—"Eye Gymnastics" – Part I, 116 – Eye Gymnastics – Part II, 117 – Oriental Medicine and Eye Health, 118 – Macrobiotic Liver Diagnosis: Your Eyes Monitor the Health of Your Largest Organ, 118 – Special Liver Cleansing and Strengthening Eye Foods, 119 – Improve Your Vision by Barefoot Walking in the Water, on the Beach or the Grass, 120 – Easy No-Routine Natural Eye Exercises—Easy Distant Vision Strengthening Exercises, 120 – Easy Exercises to Boost "Close Vision", 121 – "Easy "Peripheral Vision" Strengthening Exercise, 121 – Easy "Natural Pupil" Strengthening Exercise, 121 – How to Improve Distant Vision Using "Positive Lens" Glasses, 121 – How to Use the "Positive Lens" Glasses, 121 – The Art of Reading by William H. Bates, M.D., 123 – The Thin White Line, 123 – Ayurvedic "Nasal Wash" for Clear Vision, 123 – Chinese Taoist Secret Longevity Eye Exercise, 125 – Natural Ways to Perfect Eyesight Outline, 125 – 1. Methods of Cleansing the Eyes of Toxins, 126 – 2. Feed the Eyes, 126 – 3. Strengthening the Eye Muscles with Eye Exercises, 126 – Natural Eye Focusing Exercise, 127 – Five Minute Eye Chart Exercise Routine, 128 – Cataract Studied From an Internet Website That May Help to Improve Your Vision, 129

Chapter Eleven: Protecting and Preserving Clear Vision and Healthy Eyes, 130

– Why Do So Many People Develop Cataracts?, 131 – What Causes Cataracts, 132 – Nuclear Cataract Formation, 133 – Cortical Cataract Formation, 133 – How to Protect the Eye Lens and Overcome Cataracts, 134 – Carnosine: Positive Eye and Health Free-Radical Scavenger Supplement, 134 – Glutathione, Vitamin E, NAC and Alpha Lipoic Acid Protect the Eyes from Damage, 135 – Taurine: Maintains Optimal Function and Structure of the Eyes, 135 – Vitamin C: Protects against UV radiation and Protects the Eye Fluids, 135 – Riboflavin: Buffers Free Radicals in the Eyes, 136 – Vitamin E and Selenium: Restores Glutathione Levels, 137 – Alpha-Lipoic Acid, 137 – N-Acetyl-Cysteine and Garlic, 138 – Melatonin, 138 – Lens Protein Protection, 138 – Vitamin B6, 138 – Acetyl-L-Carnitine, 138 – Aminoguanidine, 138 – Bioflavonoids, 139 – Inositol, 139 – Ocular Environment Support, 139 – Carotenoids, Vitamin A, Astaxanthin, Lutein, Zeaxanthin: Protects the Eye Retina, 139 – Co-enzyme Q10, 139 – Potassium and Magnesium, 139 – Gingko and Bilberry, 140 – Supplemental Medicine—Overview of Ctaracts, 140 – Free Radical Reduction—Metabolic Changes and Cataract, 140 – Hydrogen Peroxide and Cataract, 140 – Metabolism Support: Key Components, 141- Protection from Free Radicals: The Glutathione Mechanism, 141 – Lens Protein Protection and Cellular Metabolism Maintenance, 141 – The Glycation Process, 142 – Maintaining a Healthy Ocular Environment, 142 – Summary, 142 – Scientific Summary, 142 – Preventing Cataracts, Glaucoma and Macula Degeneration in the First Place, 142 – Symptoms of Cataracts Formation, 143 – Cataracts come quicker if you…, 143 – Supplement Recommendations, 143 – Seven Steps to Powerful Health, 144 – Product Availability, 145 -

Chapter Twelve: The Aging Eye and Macular Degeneration: Protect Your Vision, 146

– How You Can Protect Your Vision, 146 – Age-Related Macular Degeneration (AMD), 148 – Diabetic Retinopathy, 148 – Glaucoma, 149 – Focus on Eye Health and Healthy Eating, 149 – Preventing Degernerative Eye Diseases, 150 – Reversing Diabetes and Diabetic Related Eye Diseases Through Diet and Healthy Life-Style Habits, 152 – What is a Low Insulin Index, 152 – Powerful Supplements to Optimize Your Eye Health, 153 – When Shopping for a Good Eye Formula Supplement, Lookfor These Ingredients, 153 – Health Force Research Center, Address, Phone Number, Email and Website, 154

References, 155

Appendix A: Source Page Order Products, 156
Appendix B: In Memorium, 157
Appendix C: Earthing/Grounding Barefoot Technology for Health, 161
Appendix D: Personal Health/Nutrition Coach Phone Consultations, 162
Appendix E: Amazing Pinhole Eye Glasses, 166
Appendix F: Amazing Far Infra-Red Healing Sauna Light Technology, 168
Appendix G: The Power of Astaxanthin for Health and Vision Improvement, 172
Appendix H: The Liver, Vision and Traditional Chinese Medicine (TCM, 175
Appendix I: 20 Secret Keys to Health and Longevity, 178
Appendix J: Healing Power Breath of Life: Oxygen, OxyOz Ozone Generator, 182
Index, 185
About the Authors, 189

Front Cover Picture from www.dreamstime.com

Front cover picture was chosen for its deep spiritual, physical, psychological, and symbolic meaning. If you have an "Eagle Eye," you have the vision of the Perfect Seeing Eagle. The Eagle soars high above the earth into the heavenly skies—the goal of life is to overcome or "be above" our earthly self-made problems and tribulations, and seek the Heavenly Realms, like the "All Seeing" Eagle. The Eagle is symbolic of our free spiritual nature. The Eagle is endowed with Perfect Eyesight, and can see movement below at great distances. The Eagle has All Seeing Vision, like the Sage in all of us—All Seeing Spiritual Vision. The Eagle has Perfect Eyesight because it constantly looks into the distance. We too can improve our vision by looking into the distance as much as possible during the daylight hours. The Eagle is flying toward the Golden Sun. The Golden Sun is the spiritual and physical source of all life on earth. Without the Sun, we could not have vision to see. The Eagle is symbolic of overcoming all obstacles, and by its example, we can fly high to achieve Perfect Eyesight, and all of our life goals. The Eagle is also symbolic of health and long life. In the final analysis, the cover depicts peace, calmness, tranquility, and harmony in all three aspects of life—body, mind, spirit.

Introduction

Over one-hundred million people in America have defective eyesight and that number is growing fast. Yet, very little is being done to improve the natural eyesight of Americans. Why? Natural eyesight training is not taught in schools and colleges--you have to learn it through self-study, self-effort and self- discipline, and train with a Natural Eye Trainer.

Would you like to possess perfect vision? Would you like to read fine print clearly and easily without glasses or contacts? Do you see clearly in the distance? You can if you learn to use your eyes properly. If you had normal vision as a child, there is no reason why you cannot achieve perfect eyesight now, barring serious eye scar tissue or other degenerative eye diseases.

Poor eyesight is the result of mental and physical tension, weak eye muscles, malnutrition, overeating, excessive sugar, meat, fats, protein, "junk food," excessive close eye work, lack of exercise, poor muscle tone and lack of flexibility throughout the body. Fortunately, these causes can be corrected by natural holistic health and eye methods.

Robert Zuraw suffered from advanced myopia (20-600) vision--legally termed blind without glasses. He was advised by a leading eye-specialist that his "eyesight could not be improved...come back in six months for stronger eye glasses." But, he knew deep-down inside that there must be another way to see without glasses--to achieve perfect eyesight naturally without "windowpanes", as an old American Indian once said about his 105 year old father, who could read the newspaper without "windowpanes."

The "Quest" for perfect eyesight was on. Robert Zuraw trained with a Dr. Bates' natural eye specialist in the early 1960s in Detroit. In the early 1970s, he went to Ann Arbor to learn important eye improvement techniques from Dr. Sasaki, a prominent natural eye specialist.

He searched out used and new book stores throughout the country. He learned from yogis, masters, Naturopathic and holistic health nutritional doctors. He studied German, Russian, Egyptian, Indian, African and American Natural Eyesight Systems. He absorbed and practiced every method he could find from around the world.

Today, he has good news and hope for all those suffering with poor eyesight and nowhere to turn. His eyesight is now better than "normal" 20-20-- from "blind with glasses," to "Sight Without Glasses." He has achieved his goal of "perfect eyesight." And these are words of hope and inspiration for those seeking perfect, healthy eyesight.

If you really desire perfect eyesight, then this book is for you! It outlines, in simple, step-by-step procedures, thirty years of natural eye research, condensed in an easy-to-follow program of one to two hours per week of Eye Exercises. If you practice these techniques consistently, you will soon see results.

Your eyes cannot improve by themselves; laziness and lack of effort will not improve your eyesight. However, if you are energetic, optimistic, patient and persistent—YOU WILL SUCCEED! What do you have to lose—nothing but your distorted vision.

"Vision is the most vital of the five senses. The fullest enjoyment of life comes through the eyes—the color of a flower, the form of beauty, the smile of a friend. At work, at home and at play—most of the things we do lose much of their pleasure without normal vision. You can learn to have good vision throughout life when you learn to use your eyes properly under the conditions modern life imposes upon them." --Dr. William H. Bates.

Here is something that will be worth its weight in gold to you

We have written "**Perfect Eyesight**," which represents over 35 years of study and research on improving eyesight naturally, without glasses or surgery. You don't have to suffer with poor eyesight any more! We will give you the secrets to perfect eyesight in "**Perfect Eyesight**." This book will tell you about the hidden powers latent within you to improve your vision far beyond the average. It will teach you the wonders and healing powers of the human eye, brain, nervous system and body. Why you were designed by the Creator to see "perfectly" without glasses. The book is loaded with never before revealed secrets of the eye-brain connection, and how the "**Black Box Exercise**" can improve your vision within minutes! Sounds too good to be true? Read on...

"Perfect Eyesight" will show you just what is wrong with your eyes and how to overcome poor vision—sometimes within days! "**Perfect Eyesight**" has been pronounced as priceless by thousands. Cancel your eyeglass or eye surgery appointment, until you read and practice the invaluable, result-producing information in this book. It will be a real loss to you if you do not read, understand and practice the profound secrets in "Perfect Eyesight."

"Let There Be Light"

With all our advanced technology during the last half century we have still known little about light and its greatest use—that of helping eyes to develop strong and naturally—of helping eyes to see clearly and with the minimum of effort. But now we are beginning to learn some very interesting and fundamental facts about the relation of light to sight. To appreciate its full significance however, we must first understands the conditions under which our eyes have developed.

In the beginning of the human race man was born a creature of the outdoors and his day extended only from dawn to dusk. This method of lighting continued for countless centuries, with "improvements" only in fuel oil lanterns and candles.

As civilization advanced, lighting methods advanced slowly with it. After oil lamps came gas lighting. It was not until Edison discovered how to produce light electrically within a bottle, that the world made any marked progress in lighting. Primitive man used his eyes out-of-doors under very high intensities of daylight—intensities hundreds of times greater than we find in-doors today. When the sun went down his tasks were ended for the day. He closed his eyes and went to sleep. During the day man used his eyes for distant seeing—hunting, fishing, foraging and the most menial of seeing tasks. Very little close-vision work was performed.

Even in Abraham Lincoln's time very few men or women studied or sewed or read as we do—far into the night.

Modern civilization has completely changed all this. We have lightly tossed aside the fact that our eyes were in the process of developing for hundreds of thousands of years—and developing for distance seeing under tremendous quantities of natural daylight. In the last few seconds on the clock of time we have taken liberties with all four of nature's principles:

1. Distance seeing   *2. Lots of light to aid our vision*
3. A relatively short day   *4. Easy visual tasks*

Instead, we have substituted close seeing indoors, extremely low levels of lighting, a much longer day, and abnormally severe eye-straining tasks.

The eye is a marvelous organ, but not so remarkable that it is able to adapt itself to the severe change we have imposed upon it. Perhaps that is why so much eye trouble is prevalent today. Cats can see in the dark. But your eyes and a child's eyes were never intended to do close seeing in anything but adequate light. In fact, nature developed our eyes for distant seeing, out of doors. She certainly never intended that we should use our eyes the way we do for reading books, playing games, computers, sewing or other close work, in half light. No wonder that 95% of all people over thirty years of age have impaired vision! Even 80% of grade school children have defective eyesight and require glasses or contacts. What they really need is less close work, better lighting and more outdoor activity. Certainly, something is radically wrong when we try to read or perform office work under poor light.

It is not only a matter of eye-strain. It is a matter of needlessly using up untold quantities of nervous energy. The statement has been made that the office worker who uses his or her eyes all day under inadequate light may be actually more tired at night than the man who spends all lay bricks or building a house. This indicates quite clearly that it does take energy to see. Seeing consumes energy just as definitely as shoveling snow or washing your car—even more so, because of the mental brain stress.

Suppose you drive your car for fifty miles on a bright sunny day over a straight highway. At the end of the ride you notice no particular exhaustion. But take the same car, the same road and make the same drive at night—in a fog. After fifty miles of this you know you have been doing some work. But the only difference has been the lighting. You have gripped that wheel, tensed your muscles, strained your whole body, not doing any particular work but using up a tremendous amount of nervous energy in trying to see. Shopping at a Mall, looking at all the stuff for an afternoon can leave you totally exhausted and fatigued.

Years ago, scientific studies were conducted to measure human energy consumed in the process of seeing. Dozens of people were chosen for this special laboratory test.

Each subject was seated in a comfortable chair, and asked to read page after page of a well-printed book. As he read, his hand rested on a button which he was requested to press at the end of each page. This was a means adapted for concealing the REAL purpose of the button.

What the subject did not know, however, was that he was unconsciously recording the development of nervous muscular tension produced by the reading. It was found that the average pressure unknowingly exerted upon the key was 63 grams when the reading was done under very poor light. This pressure dropped to 43 grams when the illumination was raised. In other words, the drain of nervous energy, as indicated by tension in the hand, was decreased **one-third by the use of more light.** These tests explain why poor lighting at the office or work place is a major cause of fatigue and tiredness at days end. Poor lighting and eye strain saps much of our energy.

Typists, bookkeepers, printers, mechanics and other people who use their eyes constantly for close work, are often unnecessarily fatigue before the day is over. Proper lighting will do much to ward off this fatigue and will help them accomplish their tasks with greater ease, accuracy and speed. Some interesting conclusions have been reached as a result of these tests:

The pupil of the eye becomes smaller with age; consequently, there is need for more light as we age.

If a child has to hold the book closer to his eyes than 13 or 14 inches, the probability is that he needs eyeglasses or better lighting or both.

The eyes readily adjust themselves to a variety of conditions, but will weaken under poor lighting and eye strain.

Three times as much light is required for reading a newspaper as for reading a well-printed book.

Good lighting or outdoor light helps defective eyes and prevents normal eyes from weakening. Detailed close-work, such as, sewing, watch repair, electronic repair work, surgery etc., is harder on the eyes than reading; therefore, much more light is needed.

Reading in bed is usually hard on the eyes, not only because of poor posture, but also because of inadequate and improper lighting. By correcting both conditions, the strain on the eyes is materially decreased.

Reading when the page is brightly illuminated and the rest of the room is comparatively dark often causes unnecessary eyestrain and fatigue. Some of the light should go to the walls and ceiling to bring more light in and lessen eye strain.

But, now you want to know what you can do about it. You want to know how you can light your home to conserve your eyesight and energy. The requirements for lighting the average room where most of your eye work is done would be:

1. Enough light: One or two 200 watt bulbs or full spectrum lights
2. Proper distribution of the light around the room
3. Absence of glare on the page.

Purchase a lamp that will give you direct light, without glare, and at the same time cast a reflected glow upward.

Knowledge is power. By applying the knowledge of this book, you too can improve your vision and maintain it, with clarity and power, for a lifetime.

Chapter One

The Miracle of Perfect Eyesight

The Truth About The Eyes

It is said that the eyes are the "windows" of the soul. How clear is your vision? Can you see the world without blurry vision or distortion? The so-called "normal" eye can easily read the 20 foot line on the Snellen Eye Test Chart at 20 feet away—this is called 20-20 vision. There is no limit as to how much one can improve their vision beyond the 20-20 range.

Healthy eyes are a marvel of nature's creation. A person with above average eyesight can easily read the 10 foot line (smallest bottom line on the Snellen Eye Test Chart), at 20 feet away—20-10 vision! I have seen people who can read the 10 foot line at 50 to 60 feet away—60-10 vision. This is called "telescopic vision."

There is also no limit to reading small "Microscopic Type Print"—known as "microscopic vision." There is no limit to how sharp and clear one can see in the distance and close-up. You create your own eye health, or lack thereof.

We are all walking, talking, seeing miracles of Great Nature. The sages say human beings are "solidified sunlight," or "trails of light," because our eyesight and our very life is totally dependent on the Solar Orb! We would all become blind without the healing rays of sunlight upon our retina. Sunlight also gives us natural Vitamin D for healthy skin and eyes. The eye training secrets contained in this book have taken me (Robert Zuraw), from 20-600 (progressive advanced myopia, or blindness without glasses), to better than 20-20 vision. If you practice these exercises and are persistent in your eye training, you too can improve vision over time.

Eye Muscles Accommodation: The Mystery Unveiled

In order to "see" properly, the eyes **must** accommodate. Accommodation takes place when focusing on various distances—close and far. Which muscles are doing the focusing during accommodation is debatable among Ophthalmologists. Dr. Helmholtz, an early eye doctor, found that only the "ciliary" eye muscles do the accommodating. The Helmholtz Theory is the "accepted belief" of most modern eyeglass doctors.

Dr. Bates, a natural eye specialist, felt that the two oblique eye muscles performed eye accommodation by compressing the round eyeball in the middle and making it longer horizontally. Dr. Bates cut these muscles in rabbits and found the eyes could not accommodate. When he injected a drug to paralyze the oblique muscles, the eyes failed to accommodate. When he put together the severed muscles and washed out the drug, the rabbit's eyes were able to accommodate again.

The Helmholtz theory holds that accommodation is due to the expansion and contraction of the crystalline lens, caused by the action of the ciliary muscle. Dr. Bates, through his experiments, discovered and proved that it is not the crystalline lens but the six external muscles that act upon the eyeball and give the eye its ability to adjust and accommodate to near and far objects. The fact that patients who have had the crystalline lens removed are still able to see, and have the power to accommodate, should be convincing proof of this theory.

It is obvious that both the oblique muscles and the ciliary muscles work in conjunction when focusing. Here is the reason why—the normal eye when looking at a distant object becomes shortened, and when looking at a close object is elongated.

The external muscles—oblique, recti, iris and the ciliary muscles all enable the eyes to accommodate properly. The external muscles lengthen and shorten the eyeball to enable light rays to fall upon the macula. The iris adjusts the pupil for the amount of light necessary to see clearly. And the ciliary muscle contracts the lens to focus upon the object. The ciliary muscle changes the lens and directs the rays of light to focus upon the macula or center of sight. While looking at a distant object of more than twenty feet away, the rays come into the eyes parallel. When looking at a close point rays come into the eyes at an angle.

The normal eye must accommodate these rays in order to see clearly a close or distant point. All rays from nearby objects come to a focus behind the retina. The eyes must accommodate these rays by adjusting the shape of the eye so that the rays will focus on the retina. This is accomplished by lengthening the eyeball. The oblique muscles lengthen the eyeball so the rays can focus easily on the macula. The recti muscles and the ciliary muscle work in conjunction when the eyes are focused upon a distant point, in shortening the eyeball. Simply, the external muscles focus the rays of light, the iris adjusts the light and the ciliary muscle focuses on the object

The iris adjusts the size of the pupil. In a healthy eye, the pupil is smaller when viewing a distant sight, and grows larger when seeing a close object. The pupil becomes smaller in sunlight, and grows larger when seeing a close object. The pupil becomes smaller in sunlight, and grows larger in darkness. In other words, an adjustment is made by the iris to open the pupil and let in more light to see in dim light. During a bright sunny day the iris closes the pupil—to prevent glare to see clearly. As you can readily see the iris also helps to accommodate the rays of light, so that a clear focus can be registered on the macula.

In short, the external muscles focus the rays of light, the iris adjusts the light and the ciliary muscle focuses on the object; a very simple but profound process. Eyesight is truly a miracle of nature's creation.

Weak eyesight, according to actual experience, can be corrected by strengthening the eye muscles through eye exercises, good reading habits, proper nutrition and overall improvement of health.

How Good is Your Peripheral Vision?

In the normal healthy eye peripheral vision is quite clear on the sides. Its range is very wide and high. Squinting, too much reading, heavy concentration, mental tension and malnutrition weaken the peripheral vision. The first three causes tend to center its attention on a point, while leaving out the side areas. In the Eye Exercise Technique Chapter, we will discuss a Peripheral Vision Technique to improve your side vision.

A Quick Lesson in Eye Anatomy

The First, or Sclerotic Layer is opalescent. Its center is transparent and is called thecornea. Light comes through the cornea. Behind the cornea, the second layer, orchoroid is visible.

The Second, or Choroid Layer contains tiny blood vessels which transports blood to and from the eyes.

The normal healthy eye is almost spherical and is made up of three layers of tissue: 1. The Outer Layer, or Sclerotic; 2. The Middle Layer, or Choroid; 3. The Inner Layer, or Retina. **Figure 1-1.**

Figure 1-1. The choroid layer forms in rolls around the crystalline lens and is known as the ciliary process. Located here is the ciliary muscle connected with the crystalline lens by a tiny ligament, which controls the contraction and expansion of the crystalline lens.

The Third, Inner Layer, or Retina is a continuation of the optic nerve-- located in the rear of the eye—a direct outgrowth of the brain. The retina is extremely thin and fine, and images of the outer world are cast upon it. Eyesight cannot function without the retina.

This is why good nutrition vitalizes the blood stream, and eye exercises flood the eye muscles and nerves with fresh blood and oxygen. The choroid layer contains the iris, with the pupil in its center. Right behind the iris is the crystalline lens, which absorbs light as it passes through the pupil and focuses it upon the retina.

Eye Retina's "Yellow Spot": Secret to Vision

The "Yellow Spot" is a part of the retina that allows details to enter into our vision. The center of the yellow spot is called the fovea centralis; it sees twice as good as the retina itself, particularly in bright light. When you gaze at an object or point you see with the central pit. Objects around that point are seen with the rest of the yellow spot. By focusing on an object or letter for a second or two, you see twice as well as otherwise.

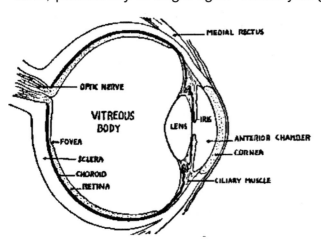

The iris adjusts the size of the pupil. The pupil, in the normal eye, when looking at a distant object is smaller.

Figure 1-1

The pupil grows larger when looking at a nearby object; it becomes smaller in sunlight and grows larger in darkness to accommodate more light. The brain and eye make an adjustment to open the pupil to let in more light to see a nearby object in dim light. During a bright sunny day the iris closes the pupil to prevent glare, so the object can be seen clearly. In the normal eye Peripheral vision is quite clear. It's side to side and up and down range is very wide and high. Squinting, too much close work and heavy long concentration weaken the Peripheral Vision. These activities actually center the eyes' attention upon a point only, while leaving out the side vision. Dr. Bates says, "The normal eye sees one thing best, but not one thing only."

Oriental Eye and Health Diagnosis

The eyes are truly the "windows of the soul' and the mirror of physical health. The human eye holds many inner secrets. Oriental herbal doctors report that the eyes operate in close connection with the liver. A poorly functioning liver causes the eyes to ache and create dark circles around them that do not bear the light very well.

Jean Rofidel, a master of Do-In (Doe-In) (Self-Massage) says: "The eyes of a person in good health bear everything: blinding light, cold and wind without crying, onions etc." If you are in good health you do not need sunglasses. "If you blink too much (more than three times a minute), it is a sign of organic weakness," (especially of the liver).

Eating too many sweets, fats, animal foods and alcohol make the eyes tired and weak. Sexual excesses causes dark circles around the eyes. Excess liquid intake causes kidney water-logging, edema, weakness, lower back pain, excess eye blinking, and puffy bags under the eyes.

How The Eyes "See"

Eyesight consists of more than the eyeball itself. It is connected to the optical apparatus, buried deep in the socket and connected to the brain itself. Rays of light converge upon the retina and forms an inverted image, which is transmitted by the optic nerve to the brain, which gives us vision. Light rays reflected from an object of vision, focus directly on the retina. However, if the eyeball is too short from front to back, light rays coming in will not focus when they hit the retina—they will diffuse or spread out, causing blurred vision. This happens because the retina is stimulated in too many places instead of at a single point. This is called farsightedness. In nearsightedness, the eyeball becomes elongated so that the light entering it are focused before they reach the retina.

Are Eye Glasses or Contacts Necessary?

When I first started natural eye training I made the mistake of throwing away my eye glasses. Discarding glasses while my eyes were still weak, actually slowed down my eye improvement for many years. Please learn from my personal experience and continue to wear glasses, especially if your vision is very weak and blurry. Straining to see without glasses too soon places excess strain and tension on the eyes and brain. Visit your local optometrist and ask for weaker lenses, or ask him to grind down your present glasses a half diopter. Vision Therapists prescribe a 20-30 lens, so that you can constantly improve your vision. As your vision fitness improves over the months and years, order weaker lenses for your glasses until you reach a point where they can be dispensed with entirely. Do not rush this process. Take enough time to strengthen your eyes with these powerful eye training methods before you discontinue using glasses.

Important Eye Note: *Full strength glasses "fix" the eyes in a permanently locked position, which cannot allow the eye muscles to focus on near or far objects. As your eyes strengthen, obtain weaker lenses from an eye glass specialist. Stronger, thick-lensed glasses always weaken the eyes.*

When your vision reaches 20-50 without glasses, you can take your glasses off without undue strain. Of course, you need to wear glasses while driving or looking into the distance. Once you are able to see 20-30 or better, you can dispense with glasses entirely. If you have close vision problems (farsightedness), wear the weakest lens that still enables you to see the print. Gradually, have the lens weakened until you no longer need glasses to perform close work or reading.

Eye glasses and 'contacts' are at best a "crutch" for the eyes; they do not halt poor vision or stop the cause of faulty vision. We need to look for the individual cause or causes of weak vision. The cause can usually be found in poor eye habits, poor nutrition, excessive eye straining, close work etc.

Important Eye Note: Seventy-five percent of Americans are vision impaired! How would you like to be among the 25% with strong sharp vision? You can. You are the only one who can improve your vision. If you follow these eye instructions faithfully and persistently, your eyes WILL improve.

At odd times during the day, remove your glasses to accustom your eyes to see naturally without them. If you practice these eye training routines with patience, determination and dedication, you too may soon have perfect sight without glasses. Stick to it! You must give it time.

In **Chapter Two**, we'll discuss the importance of **'Daily Eye Strengthening Habits.'** These easy to perform "Habits" can be performed throughout the day, i.e., waiting in line at the store, driving, stopped in traffic, or even while reading, watching television, walking etc. They are enjoyable to do, and will extend your clear vision well into advanced age. Read on, and enjoy your quest for Perfect Eyesight.

How Long Does It Take to Achieve 20-20 Vision?

Working with natural eye training methods takes time. Everyone has different eye conditions. It all depends on how poor your vision is. How long you have worn glasses or contacts? If you thoroughly understand and apply these natural eye teachings, your vision will improve at a faster pace.

If your vision is 20-50 or less, it may take a few weeks to a few months to bring your vision back to normal (20-20). If you have 20-70 to 20-100 vision, it may take several months to a year. If you have 20-200 or worse, it may take a few years. It all depends on your understanding, dedication and consistent practice of these special eye training techniques.

No matter how long it takes, the goal is to become naturally visually fit. Most people after the age of 45 require glasses and begin losing their vision. You will not lose your vision if you perform these exercises conscientiously, even into advanced age once you acquire normal 20-20 vision. If you consult with a Natural Vision Instructor your eyesight will improve faster, because they will show you how to relax your mind, body and eyes.

Knowledge and Wisdom Bring Understanding and Practice

IMPORTANT EYE TRAINING NOTE: *When you understand how the eye functions, you will practice the eye exercises with knowledge and insight. The eye is an intricate organ of the body, connected to the brain, nervous system, liver and bloodstream, and can be strengthened and rejuvenated just as the body. Eyesight is a marvelous miracle of creation. If the eyes are not abused they will take care of you for a long, healthy and happy life. A toxic, congested liver, cells and tissues can cause eye problems.*

Chapter Two

Daily Eye Strengthening Habits

Practice Distance Seeing

The human eye was not designed for extended use in close-work (reading, computers, factory work, sewing etc). Gazing into the distance is the natural position of the eye (20 or more feet away). Ciliary eye muscles RELAX when viewing objects more than 20 feet away because the rays of light come in parallel. During close-work, light flows into the eyes diversely, thus causing ciliary eye muscle strain, because it must "contract" to allow light to focus upon the macula.

Myopia (nearsightedness) has two causes: 1. Not focusing or using the eyes enough while looking into the distance; 2. Performing excessive close- work.

Unfortunately, we live in a close-vision world. Twenty-first century life has reduced the need for clear, far-seeing eyesight. Many people rarely look at an object more than 50 feet away. Excessive close-work has caused an epidemic of weak distant vision.

Books, magazines, newspapers, precision work in our offices, factories and schools require extreme close-vision for hours at a time. Our eyes were simply not designed for this constant close-work. Most of us start out in life with good vision, but after high school and college and years in front of a computer, we end-up with "thick-window-pane-glasses." Our health and vision deteriorate in spite of our material knowledge and credentials. We need wisdom with knowledge to give us true understanding of how the eyes truly function.

Do you want clear, sharp vision? Then you must practice distance-seeing.Practice distance-gazing while walking, lunch breaks—look out the window into the distance to distinguish objects at or slightly beyond the far-limits of what you can see now. This practice helps to push back this limit to see further. Remember to always focus on objects you can see and strive to bring them into clearer focus. Relax your gaze. Never strain. Read distant signs, distinguish license plate numbers of passing cars. Watch birds in flight. Look at distant airplanes. Count stars at night.

What Causes Weak Eye Muscles?

Tests on thousands of people over the years have proven beyond doubt that in most cases weak vision is caused by strain on the eye muscles. Eye strain causes tense eye-muscles; tense muscles connected to the eyeball, eventually distort the shape of the eye. This is a fundamental principle in eye improvement training: By relaxing the tension in the eye muscles and strengthening weak eye muscles, weak or defective eyes can definitely be made strong again.

Myopia, or **nearsightedness** means that the eyeball is **elongated;** and **farsightedness** hypermetropia) and presbyopia (old age sight) means that the eyeball is **flattened**. This is caused by defective accommodation, which is caused by weak, unbalanced eye muscles. A myopic eye is "frozen" in an elongated position, making it hard to see objects in the **distance.** The farsighted eye is "frozen" in a flat position, making it hard to see **near objects.**

The liver sends energy, nerve impulses and blood to the eyes. Therefore, a clean blood stream, and a healthy functioning liver, which heals and strengthens the eyes. However, if the colon and liver is toxic and blocked with wastes, the blood becomes impure, health declines, and eyes will become weak, drab, with heavy dark circles around them. Eyes cannot be treated as an unconnected isolated organ. The blood stream and nervous system is directly connected to the eyes. There is an intimate association between the liver, blood and eyes. When the body cells and liver becomes weak, toxic and unhealthy, the eyes reflect this weakened condition.

Do you want healthy vibrant eyes? Then you must build up your health and vitality through diet, exercise and eye training methods. Of prime importance is wholesome, unprocessed foods and thorough bowel elimination, two to three times a day.

Look Up From Your Close Work

This is an important eye habit you can practice while reading, at the office or watching television. It helps the eyes from getting into a frozen position. Simply look UP from your close-work every five minutes and gaze (focus) at a distant object for five seconds. This exercise prevents eye-muscle cramping and also relaxes the eye muscles.

Natural eye doctors, Drs. Ross and Rehner advise us to "Look up and away from your close work at frequent intervals. No matter how fascinating or important your reading, drawing, or sewing may be, glance away from it for a few seconds every 5 minutes. This is just as important, as it is simple to do. We want you to continue this even when your sight has returned to normal."

During close work, the ciliary muscles contract to properly focus the lens. These muscles kept in constant contraction for long periods, tend to remain cramped, thus when looking up, the vision becomes fuzzy. Holding a barbell in a fully flexed arm curl position for several minutes, causes the biceps and fingers to cramp strongly. When the weight is put down, the fingers take a minute to "uncurl" themselves from their tight contracted grip on the bar. The biceps also remains tight and contracted momentarily.

This same principle applies to the eye muscles. Too much close-work cramps the eye muscles in one position and keeps them there if the "cramping" is not discontinued. The practice of looking up every few minutes minimizes eye muscle cramping, which causes the eyes to be focused for the near point when we wish to see farther away.

Avoid Close Work During and After Meals

Dr. Sasaki, a Japanese Eyesight Specialist states that you can add twenty years to your life if you do not read while eating, and go outdoors after meals for at least 30 to 60 minutes. Why does reading and close-work during and after meals impair the eyesight? Close work draws blood to the eyes, instead of being used for digestion, thus causing lack of nutrients to the eyes, weak eye muscles and cloudy vision.

Going outside after meals provides the necessary oxygen to properly digest and assimilate food. Spending one hour outdoors after meals vastly enhances digestive powers, which improves and strengthens eyesight. Humans require large amounts of outdoor oxygen, especially for the kidneys, liver and eyes. This imparts vigorous health and superior eyesight. Breathing in outdoor oxygen and performing deep breathing exercises in the fresh outdoor air helps in the production of healthy red blood cells; it improves cellular oxygen; and it gives us inspiration, good health and long life. Take advantage of the outdoors often, especially in warm, sunny weather.

Fourteen Eye Habits For Perfect Eyesight

Eye Habit Number One
Do not read when tired or sick

The body is a flowing, dynamic energy machine operating on Chi-Energy--Cosmic Chi, Earthly Chi and Food Chi. When the body is ill or tired, the eyes also become tired and blurry. Weak bodily energy weakens the entire system, especially the Liver, which is directly connected to the eyes via the acupuncture meridians. Reading during illness or fatigue weakens the focusing eye muscles.

Do you remember a past illness or stress situation you had? You can bet your eyesight became dim or cloudy during that period. In my teens I did plenty of reading late at night when I could scarcely keep my eyes open; this was a great strain on my eyes. Consequently, my eyesight weakened. The rule of thumb here is to read or perform close work when your energy is high; during illness or fatigue obtain plenty of rest and sleep.

> **_Important Health Note_:** The body, mind and eyes heal and rejuvenate during rest and a good solid night's sleep. Lack of sufficient rest and sleep can easily run down your immune system--liver, gastrointestinal system, and result in poor vision.

Refrain from reading in poor lighting. Nature, or outside solar light, gives us 10,000 watts of bright light. Inside lighting is very dim in comparison, seldom reaching 150-200 watts. Most people read with 60-100 watt bulbs or less and strain their eyes. If you have trouble reading in dim light, your eyes will strain and weaken even more.

It is best to read in daylight, with the sun or outdoor light coming through the window onto your reading or working material. Or better yet, do your reading or close work outdoors when the weather is clear and pleasant. When night-time approaches, make sure you shine a bright bulb—150-200 watts—onto your reading material to make it clear, and lessen eye strain. Adjust the light so it does not cause a glare on the page. Dr. Vogel recommends not to read at night before bed or in bed, as this can further weaken vision, cause bloodshot eyes, fatigue and insomnia.

Maintain a good posture while reading. Poor posture while reading is a major cause of weakened and fatigued eyesight. Avoid slumping or hanging or craning your head down while reading. Sit comfortably erect. A slumped head position causes the eyes to point downward. This causes gravity to pull down on the eyeballs, which places strain on the extrinsic eye muscles, while holding the eyes back in the sockets. Holding this 'neck-bent downward position' causes lengthening of the eyeball, resulting in myopia or nearsightedness (flattening of the eyeball).

Hold print parallel twenty inches from the eyes. Please understand: holding the print to close to the eyes is a *major* cause of myopia. When I observe young people holding their reading material too close to their eyes (less than 10"), I know they are heading for myopic vision. Dr. Sasaki and many other natural eye doctors do not recommend excessive reading for youngsters; read only when necessary. They need to gaze into the distance as often a possible. Many myopics can improve their sight by this one important eye habit.

Eye Habit Number Two
Do not read more than thirty minutes at a time

Thirty minutes is about maximum time the eyes can handle without strain or fatigue. Read for awhile, then get up and walk around, stretch or go outside for a breath of fresh air. Look into the distance. Take a deep breath, bend over and rub your face, forehead and around the eyes, exhale and stand straight. Inhale again and bend backward, then to each side, and exhale and relax your gaze. Close your eyes and place your palms over your eye sockets; think or visualize black velvet or a large black dot. This palming method was taught by Dr. Bates. Deep breathing, face and head rubbing, bending and twisting and palming all help to refresh the brain and eyes, imparting increased energy and clear thinking. Make it your 'refreshment' break instead of coffee or pop.

Strain is the major cause of imperfect eyesight. Straining to "see" any object, far or near, in which you are enable to see clearly, places a heavy strain on the eye muscles. Similarly, straining to lift a heavy weight can strain a tendon or muscle. Straining to read fine print in poor lighting causes weak vision at the close point (farsightedness).

Holding the print too close (less than 12 inches), reading excessively, and straining to "make out" objects in the distance is the major cause of nearsightedness (myopia). The correct method to read and avoid farsighted vision is to: 1) Read in good bright light; 2) While reading or performing close work, every few minutes focus in on a letter on the page, and gaze at it for five to ten seconds.

To help overcome myopia, look into the distance at an object you can "see clearly" for a few seconds; this helps one to regain distance vision if it is weak or blurry. It is important to **not** gaze at objects you cannot see well enough—this strains the eyes even more! Practice looking at things effortlessly and relaxed. If you cannot 'see' an object clearly, do not strain to see it. Either get closer to the object, use brighter lighting, or temporarily wear glasses.

Here are a few other causes of eye strain: Long exposure to cold wind in the eyes and bright artificial lights, (especially fluorescent lights). Watching television or movies excessively strains tired weak eyes. To strengthen, heal and relax your tired and strained eyes look at nature's outdoor bounties: green trees, green grass, mountains, beautiful flowers, flowing rivers, blue-green oceans, the open sky, the stars at night, the moon, the sun at sunrise or sunset—nature herself. She is the only one who can heal you, with the help of healing chi energy from the heavens.

Eye Habit Number Three
The Invigorating Lemon Juice Eye Bath

Dr. William Apt, a leading eye specialist in the mid-1900s, recommended the Lemon Juice Eye Bath. He stumbled upon this secret from a 105 year old man. He instructed Dr. Apt to "put three or four drops of lemon juice in an eye cup with purified water and wash the eyes with it daily for about 20-30 seconds with each eye." Dr. Apt says it is invigorating and strengthening. It removes toxic fatigue of the eye. This ancient oldster washes his eyes daily, eats natural foods, wears no glasses, and has perfect eyesight!. The Lemon Juice Eye Bath is also recommended to cure cataracts, with osteopathic treatment, plus a strict seven-day elimination (vegetable and fruit) diet, once a month.

Perfect Eyesight

The continuous practice of these Zuraw Eye Training Techniques will eventually help you to **see clearly** what you cannot see now.

Eye Habit Number Four
Healing Sun Part I: Sunshine is Food for the Eyes

Sunlight is "food" for the eyes. It thrives on it. It is nourished and healed by its warm radiating energy. Go outdoors in the sunlight everyday—walk when you can, work in the garden, read a book, gaze into the distance, enjoy sports—whatever you enjoy, do more of it in the life-giving sun and fresh air. Coal miners have observed that mules kept in a dark coal mine, eventually lose their sight.

The best time to enjoy the sunshine is in the morning before 11:00 am or after 3:00 pm. Nature's Sun produces 10,000 watts of natural light; indoor bulbs are a weak 100 watts in comparison. One of the major causes of poor eyesight in this so-called "modern society" is staying indoors during daylight hours. Human thrive on outdoor oxygen and sun light. We live on a carbon based planet, filled with oxygen and solar light. This is our human biological destiny.

The human body was designed by nature to be an outdoor dweller most of the time. We have switched our position in the scheme of things and fallen prey to our own arrogance and ignorance. We are the ones who suffer from lack of sun and air. Nature is there waiting for us to partake of her fragrance, beauty and bounty.

Outdoor people generally have better vision than indoor dwellers. The famous old-time lion tamer, Johnny Pack, enjoys several hours a day of sunshine, and at 91 years young in 1996, has excellent eyesight at both far and close point.

Healing Sun Part II: Sunshine is Food for the Eyes
Secrets of Yoga Sun Gazing

How would you like to possess magnetic healthy eyes? Develop a steady powerful gaze? Approach life situations without fear? The ancient Yogis use this as a meditation technique and to infuse the body, mind and spirit with light and power.

How to Perform the Yoga Sun Gazing Exercise: Go outside at SUNRISE or SUNSET when the orb is red or orange. Open your eyes wide and take in 9 deep breaths (in and out gently) while looking at the sun. Feel the "sun energy" traveling into your eyes and down to your belly button area (Hara). After sun gazing, gently cover your eyes with your palms for a few minutes while visualizing the color black. This helps to relax and heal stress and tension in the
mind and eyes.

Acquire plenty of sunshine, allowing fresh air to hit your bare skin and walking on the earth with bare feet all help to improve our eyesight. Practice these golden treasures whenever possible. The Immortal Taoist Masters cherish these activities, along with Chi Kung Exercises, as the keys to health, energy and longevity.

Healing Sun Part III: Sunshine is Food for the Eyes
Sunglasses Harmful?

Sunglasses shield our eyes from the life-giving sun. Wearing sun glasses constantly can lead to photo-phobia (fear of light), or light sensitivity. Some eye specialists warn against the excessive use of sunglasses. They report that it can cause blindness by paralyzing the eye-pupil.

In bright light the pupil becomes smaller and in darkness it becomes larger. Wearing sunglasses in sunlight keeps the pupil expanded because the shaded lens does not allow light to enter. This is what weakens our eyes. If you are driving into the sunset or sunrise, use your sunglasses to reduce glare, otherwise leave them off. You can also purchase Dr. Ott's Full Spectrum sun glasses. They take out the sun glare and let in beneficial light rays.

If the sun bothers your eyes, the best remedy is to spend more time out-of-doors in the daylight and secondly, consume a better diet consisting of whole grains, vegetables, fruits, seeds and protein for your individual body type. (See Body Typing Chapter). One of the greatest foods for the eyes is sunflower seeds and parsley. They contain Vitamin B-2, which helps to overcome light sensitivity. If you avoid the sun completely, you'll become over-sensitive to even 10 minutes of it. Get some sun, within reason.

Morning or early evening sun is the best time for sunbathing. On hot days, walk in the shade and gaze into the distance. You will soon adjust to the light and even enjoy it. Well sunned eyes glow with magnetism and health.

Eye Habit Number Five
The Oriental 'Yang Eye' Candle Gazing Technique

This powerful Yang Eye Candle Gazing Technique has been taught and practiced in the East for thousands of years. It is known to give one glowing magnetic eyes. You can look at anyone in the eye without fear or timidity.

This "Yang Eye" Technique not only improves the eyesight, but is known by the ancient Taoist masters to alleviate many eye problems, and latent ailments within the body. The whites of the eyes will become clear, and your eyes will shine with brightness.

How to Perform the "Yang Eye Candle Gazing Technique: Light a candle and sit in front of it at arms length and at eye level. Gaze steadily at it without blinking. Breathe naturally, and continue gazing for five minutes without moving your body. Try not to move your eyelids. Less movement brings more magnetic power and control into the eyes and nervous system.

Keep your eyes open and allow the tears to flow down your cheeks; open your eyes wider as the tears flow down. Every minute or so, close your eyes for 10 or 15 seconds. Finish by closing your eyes and palming for two minutes to cool-down your eyes.

Perfect Eyesight

Eye Habit Number Six
The East Indian Yoga Nasal Massage Technique

Ayurvedic East Indian Medicine teaches us that chronic colds, flu, mucus and lung congestion is the basic cause of most eye problems. The eyes are in close proximity to the nasal and sinus passages.

Nasal massage helps to improve sinus conditions and allows you to see objects with clarity. It also helps to relieve emotional tension, which builds up in the face, forehead and eyes. We tense our face when under stress.

How to Perform the Yoga Nasal Massage Technique: Dip your baby finger into sesame oil, or use one drop of eucalyptus oil and insert it into each nostril and massageas deep as possible. Slowly massage in a clockwise and counterclockwise direction. You may feel soreness. Go easy. You may also sneeze and blow your nose several times. Don't panic. This is a 'cleansing action' by your body. It'll clear your sinuses pronto! It opens up the lung-breathing channels, releases pent-up emotions, and improve eye clarity. Gently massage the inside nose tissue each morning before breakfast at least 3 times a week.

Eye Habit Number Seven
Chinese Taoist Kidney, Stomach & Liver Massage
Note: This is the Key to Super-Health and Clear-Vision

The kidneys, stomach and liver are reflex organs to the ears, mouth and eyes. In Chinese Medicine, the kidneys are considered the health and longevity organs of the body. Weaken the kidneys and the health of the entire body begins to fail. The stomach is considered the central energy station or grand central station for food distribution to the entire system. The Liver is the great detoxifying organ of the body. It filters out chemicals, pollutants, preservatives, fats, oils etc. Overeating any type of fats, even good oils, nuts, nut butters, avocados, can easily congest and weaken the liver and vision. A weak liver places great stress on the immune system. Congestion in the liver causes poor food digestion, fatigue and can easily lead to yeast infections, PMS and blood disorders. These internal organ massage techniques, performed regularly, can help improve vision and increase overall health.

How to Perform the Kidney Massage. Rub your hands together until hot and place them over the kidneys (right and left side of lower back) for 10 seconds. Next, rub the kidney area vigorously, at least 35 times up and down. Finish by lightly pounding the kidney area with your palms.

How to Perform the Stomach and Liver Massage: Rub under right and left side of rib cage 35 times. The liver is under the right rib cage. The stomach is under the left rib cage. This Dao-In massage can help sharpen your vision and bring energy and healing power into your stomach and liver.

Perfect Eyesight

Eye Habit Number Eight
Acupressure Eye Massage and Eye Palming Techniques

Acupressure has been around for thousands of years, introduced to the West by the Chinese Acupuncture Masters. Acupressure is finger pressure therapy on meridian points or pathways that run up and down the body, arms, legs, head and face.

How to Perform the Acupressure Eye Massage Technique: Exert heavy finger pressure upon each of the points surrounding the eyes for 10 seconds. Next, rub each point for 5 seconds. See **Figure 1-2**. Any pain denotes eye weakness. Healthy eyes have no pain, even under heavy finger pressure. If your eyes are very weak, spend more time on eye massage. Next, with the pads of the first 3 finger tips, press lightly upon closed eye lids for 30 seconds—this helps myopia (nearsightedness).

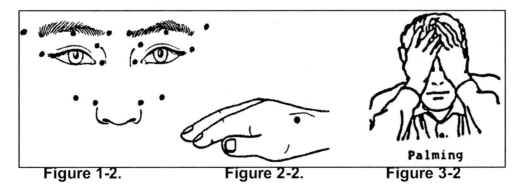

Figure 1-2.   **Figure 2-2.**   **Figure 3-2**

Figure 2-2. Locate the hoku point on each hand and massage each hand for 30 seconds.

Finish with the Eye Palming Technique: Rub hands together until hot and place cupped palms over both eyes for 30 seconds. Visualize dark black velvet—it is very relaxing. Perform Eye Palming daily; it is restful and healing for the eyes, mind and entire body. **Figure 3-2**.

Eye Habit Number Nine
Powerful Neck Loosening Exercises

Tenseness around the neck and shoulders can cause severe eye tension. To loosen-up your neck and release tension perform **Neck Rolls (Figure 4-2)** as follows: a) turn your head in a circular motion; b) move it left to right as far as you can; and c) let it drop forward and then backward as far as possible; while head is all the way back; lift both shoulders up and near your earlobes and move head right to left and left to right several times. This movement squeezes the tension right out of the neck and trapezious muscles.

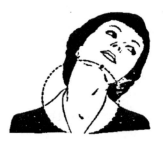

Figure 4-2

Perfect Eyesight

You will feel relaxed and refreshed after performing this movement for one to two minutes. Do these exercises often during the day; it will help to reduce eye strain, neck tightness and eye tension headaches.

Eye Habit Number Ten
Taoist Dao-Yin Eye Massage Techniques

Oriental Taoist and Zen masters practice a form of self-healing massage called Do-In (Dao-Yin). Dao-Yin is a chi-energy technique, which combines with Chi Kung breathing movements to revive and regenerate the body, mind, emotions and spirit, harmonizing all levels of being with the rhythm of life. Dao-Yin, practiced daily helps one to maintain balance and harmony in life. It helps keep one centered, grounded and focused in life.

Eye Massage Technique A
Chinese Scalp Rubbing Eye Technique

Sit straight and relax mind and body. Simply rub your scalp with fingers slowly from front to back and in small circles for 30 to 60 seconds. (**Figure 5-2**). This helps to clear the heart of toxins, relax the brain, calm nerves, invigorate the scalp and improve eyesight by bringing blood circulation to the head and eye region. Scalp massage reduces tension and stress. Even better, exchange scalp massage with your friend. It's even more relaxing and soothing when someone else does it for you.

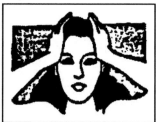

Figure 5-2

Eye Massage Technique B
Palm Eye Massage Technique

Close eyes slightly and knead closed eye-lids over eyeballs with the inside of your palms. (**Figure 6-2**). Circle palms 16 times clockwise and 16 times counterclockwise. Next, place palms on the eyes and move up and down 16 times, and side to side 16 times. This is, from my experience, the best eye massage for all conditions: Nearsightedness, farsightedness, astigmatism and helps to prevent eye diseases of the middle-aged and elderly. (Location of eye kneading)

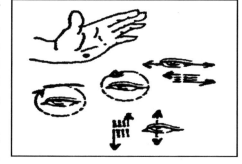

Figure 6-2

Eye Massage Technique C
Stroking Eyebrows Technique
Place thumbs on temple and stroke eyebrows with second knuckle of each forefinger, over eyebrows. Rub 16 times. Close eyes and use light and even pressure. This helps to clear the eyes, regulate nerve function, prevents hardening of cerebral arteries, and degenerative eye diseases.

Eye Massage Technique D
Ironing the Face Technique
Scrub the face with open palms from the forehead, down to the chin, and up to the ears in a circular motion, 16 times. The Chinese Taoists' call this "Ironing the Face." It helps to remove wrinkles, brings fresh blood to the eyes and improves one's complexion.

Eye Habit Number Eleven
Squeeze Eyes Tightly and Open Eyes Widely
Breathe in slowly and gradually squeeze your eyes tightly for 10 to 15 seconds. Next, slowly exhale, making the sound "ssshhh" while opening your eyes widely. Repeat 3-6 times. This Taoist eye technique increases circulation to the eyes, prevents watery eyes, strengthens the eyelids and tear gland muscle (orbiculairs palpebrarum), which normalizes the lachrymal glands. These glands furnish an alkaline solution that purifies the eyes and imparts a brilliant, sparkling luster to the eyes.

The Chi Kung Healing Sound "Ssshhh" is used to purify the liver and calm the nervous system. Opening the eye wide while exhaling the sound "ssshhh" releases anger and tension from the liver and the eyes.

Eye Habit Number Twelve
Naturopathic Eye Massage Technique
Naturopathic eye massage technique was used in the 1800s by Naturopathic doctors, Health and Physical Culture practitioners to improve eyesight and prevent vision problems. Follow these steps:

Step 1. Place the palm of each hand on the bony ridge above each eye. Press hard on the brow and move the skin up-and-down, side-to-side and in small circles. Perform twelve times with each area.

Step 2. Place your open palms on each side of your temples. Move the skin up and down, forward and back and in a circular motion a dozen times each.

Step 3. Place your fingers on each cheekbone under the eyes, while moving the skin up and down, right and left, a dozen or more times each.

"If you faithfully carry these instructions out it will prove of great importance in restoring your vision." Edmund Shaftsbury

Eye Habit Number Thirteen
Tracking or Edging: The Secret to Crystal Sharp Vision

How would you like to possess crystal sharp vision? Would you like to keep your vision when you are 50, 60, 70 and beyond? You can, if you faithfully follow and practice the techniques in this book.

We are told that when we reach 40 years of age or more, we will lose the ability to focus at the close point, because the aging process produces a thickening in the lens of the eyes. Yet, myopics over the age of seventy can read fine print up close easily. How do the "experts" explain that? The truth is that the reason we lose our close vision and distant vision is because we have never learned, or we have forgotten the habit of focusing. Dr. Bates called this "Central Fixation." Modern pioneers in vision training refer to it as 'tracking.' (edging- tracing). When you lose the ability to focus, you tend to peer hard, staring fixedly and forcing yourself to see, or squinting the eyes. These bad eye habits will impair your eyes even further.

In order to see clearly, the ray of light must focus directly on the macula. In the center of the macula there is a tiny depression known as the Fovea. Our best vision comes when the rays of light focus directly into the macula area.

How to Perform The Tracking Eye Technique: Tracking or Edging helps one to regain the natural ability to focus upon the macula. To improve your distant vision, 'Edge' or 'Trace' your eyes around a picture or a large letter on a sign that you can see clearly. Edge or Track around a table in the distance. As you practice edging, objects become sharp and clear to you. Practice outdoors! Sunlight makes everything more clear. Look up and down buildings, billboards, highway signs. Edge or Track along window frames, houses, trees; use your imagination. You can also use your nose as a focal point while edging; this relaxes the head and neck; this prevents the eyes from staring with a fixed gaze.

To improve your close vision, Track letters on the printed page. Each week pick out smaller and smaller letters until you can read the smallest print easily. Remember to close your eyes for a few moments between Tracking or Edging.

Point your nose at an object you have chosen and move the tip of the nose along its edges. At first, move slowly around the object, seeing each part of the Edge. Later as you become proficient, you can speed up the Edging.

You can also Track by moving your eyes only around any object, i.e., house, tree etc., or letter on a page. Remember to breathe deeply and easily while Tracking. Tracking can be done anytime, i.e., while walking, looking out the window, reading etc. Close your eyes after Tracking to rest them. Tracking can also be done with your eyes closed,

Perfect Eyesight

by mentally remembering the object. If you are seeking super-sharp vision, practice **Tracking** frequently.

> ***Important Vision Training Note:*** **"Tracking" is one of the most important eye improvement secrets I have discovered in thirty years of research in my quest for Perfect Eyesight.**

Eye Habit Number Fourteen
Head Lift Technique for Eye and Ear Problems

The "Head Lift" Technique is an excellent result-producing exercise to clear up ear and eye problems. It also helps to overcome headaches, neck and shoulder pain.

How to perform the Head Lift Technique: Place entire hand--fingers and palms around the neck at the lower part of the skull (mastoid protuberance). Next, lift your head upward and a bit forward, while turning your head to the right as you are lifting. Next, turn and lift head to the left in the same manner. This simple movement can help unblock any pinched nerves in the neck or trapezius muscles, which are attached to the neck. Lift up your head gently, but do not squeeze the neck too hard. Turn as far as you can, comfortably, in each direction, without straining or jerking. Practice the "Head Lift" several times daily, especially before sleep.

Note: Neck and shoulder massage: It is also a good idea to practice Do-In (Dao Yin) or Self-Massage to your neck and shoulders, with your fingers, knuckles and palms. If you have any soreness or energy blockages in these areas, by massaging them, you will feel renewed energy and fresh blood flowing to your head, brain and eyes. Without the proper nerve and blood supply to the eyes, vision improvement cannot progress at a steady rate. In fact, nerve and blood flow blockages can definitely hold back your quest for Perfect Eyesight. For faster eyesight improvement, the "Head Lift" Technique is unsurpassed.

> **Important Eye Note:** Myopics (nearsighted people) attempt to see a whole object, i.e., car, building etc., at once. Those with poor close vision (farsighted) attempt to see a whole page. Keep in mind that the eyes can only see one part best for clear sharp vision

In the next chapter we will discuss and outline a **"Perfect Eyesight Exercise Program"** for nearsightedness and farsightedness. This will help you to improve your vision, or to maintain and prevent further vision problems. Turn the page to **Chapter Three**, and get ready to embark on a quest for "Perfect Eyesight."

Chapter Three

Perfect Eyesight Exercise Techniques

Eyes need exercise just as much as other muscles. If you place your arm in a brace for a few weeks it starts to atrophy or get weaker and smaller; the blood cannot circulate sufficiently to impart strength and growth to the arm muscles. The eyes also have tiny muscles called 'ciliary' eye muscles that pull the eyes in all directions. When eye muscles get weak, vision becomes unfocused and our eyesight weakens. The eye muscles have lost their power to focus the eyeball itself on a close or distant point. Myopic(nearsightedness) or presbyopia (farsightedness) is a result of weak eye muscles.

We need to flex our eye muscles. Perform sets and reps of exercises to bring them back into focus. Eyes need to "pump iron" and show off their strength. Eye muscles can be strengthened to see telescopically. What others' can see with binoculars, a person with 'telescopic vision' can see without them! That's considered 'super-vision-- far above the average. But it takes some work, persistence and perseverance. However, it can be fun and enjoyable if you do it with a happy, positive attitude. Take your time; no rushing; calm your mind; turn the phone off. Focus your mind on the exercises; block out all distractions, mentally and physically. You can do it with persistence and patience.

Eye Exercise Protocol

Practice these eye exercise techniques two or three times a week. Take one, two or three day rest between each eye session, depending on your energy level. The day after your first eye routine your eye muscles may be sore; do not worry, this "soreness" will gradually leave. Soreness means that you have "exercised" weak eye muscles lying dormant for many years. They are resilient, and like your biceps arm muscle, will respond with renewed vigor. The rest period between each eye exercise session is as important as the eye exercises. During periods of rest the eyes and body heals and rebuilds, imparting strength and health. Performing eye exercises too often can easily cause eye strain, which is a basic reason why most eye routines fail.

Never wear glasses while performing eye exercises. If you are able to move around without your glasses, do so when you start this program; otherwise wear them after your eye session during your daily activities. As your eyesight improves visit your eye doctor to be fitted for weaker eye glass lenses. Be persistent and your vision will improve.

"Lazy Eight" Neck Loosening Exercise
(Pre-Eye Exercise Warm-Up Technique)

Performing the lazy eight exercise slowly and smoothly loosens the back of the neck, calms the nervous system, and enables you to focus your eyes clearly. Simply draw imaginary "eights" with your nose. Large "figure-eights" drawn with your nose helps to relax the larger muscles of the eyes, while tiny "figure eights" relax the smaller muscles of the eyes.

How to Perform Lazy Eight Exercise: Draw figure-eights with your nose; move your head slowly and smoothly. Vary the "figure eights" by drawing them vertically, then horizontally. Draw large ones and finally tiny "figure eights." Perform them in both directions--right to left and left to right; top to bottom and bottom to top. Spend at least three minutes on this exercise.

The **Lazy Eight Neck Exercise** is performed first in your routine because it relaxes your neck muscles and allows fresh blood to flow to the eyes and brain. It prepares you for the rest of your eye routine and insures greater success in improving your vision. The Eye Exercises that follow, if practiced regularly and consistently, can help bring your vision back to 20-20 and beyond! Perform the Eye Exercises with joy and relaxation. Results will be forthcoming.

Eye Exercise One
Egyptian Black Dot Technique - Part I
(Eye Muscle Exercise)

The **Egyptian Black Dot Technique** is one of the most important exercises for all eye conditions. Note: If you have trouble seeing close (farsightedness) do not perform this first part of the Black Dot Technique. Perform the second part only below.

Draw a Black Dot about the size of a dime on a 2"x3" card with black ink. Hold the card in front of your eyes, keeping your head steady. **Figure 1-3.** Next, move card to the tip of your nose and gaze at the black dot for 30 seconds.

How to Perform the Egyptian Black Dot Technique: You must see only one dot. (Figure1-3). If you see two dots, move the card away from the nose until you see one dot. After 30 seconds move the card straight out in front of your eyes, then rest and close your eyes for a few seconds. Next, raise the card up between your eyebrows and gaze at the dot for 30 seconds. Move the card as close as you can while seeing only one dot. Rest for a few seconds.

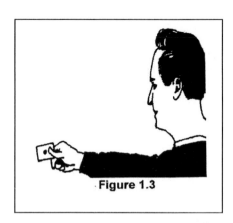
Figure 1.3

Be sure that you only see one dot; this means that both eyes are working together. Be persistent and consistent and you will see results. Remember to breathe gently, deeply and naturally.

Egyptian Black Dot Technique - Part II

While keeping the head straight, move the black dot to your right shoulder and gaze at it for 30 seconds. Then, move dot to your left shoulder and gaze at it for 30 seconds. Close eyes and rest. Farsighted people can perform this shoulder to shoulder Black Dot Exercise with great benefit. The Black Dot Techniques make the eye muscles focus in positions it does not normally focus in. This helps to reshape and balance the eyeball itself.

Eye Exercise Two
Egyptian Letter Gazing Technique - Part I
(Eye Muscle Exercise for Close and Distant Vision)

Cut out three 1/8" to 1/4" thick letters from a newspaper or magazine and glue them on a 2 x 3 white card. **Figure 2-3.** Perform each exercise with one eye at a time, then both eyes together. The eye that is covered with your palm is to be kept **open** during the exercise. This enables both eyes to work together during the exercise. Start out with three repetitions in each direction. Every two to three weeks ad one repetition, until you reach six.

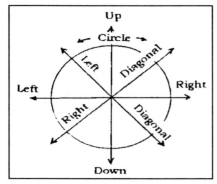
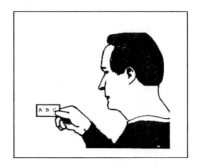

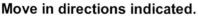

Move in directions indicated.   Figure 2-3. Egyptian Black Letter Exercise

First Movement: Hold the card twelve inches in front of your eyes. Concentrate on one of the letters, always focusing to see it clearly. Move the card above the eyes and below the chin three times. Do this one eye at a time and then both eyes together. Keep your head still—move your eyes only.

Second Movement: Hold card twelve inches in front of your eyes. Move the card slowly from your right eye to your left eye—always keeping sight of the letter. Perform with one eye, then both eyes together, three times each.

Third Movement: Hold the letter in front of your face, and move the card in right and left diagonally. Perform three times each way. Again, one eye at a time, then both together.

Fourth Movement: Move card in large circles, at arms length. Perform three times each way, one eye at a time, then both together.

Fifth Movement: Hold the card about one foot in front of your head and move the card smoothly in a ten inch diameter circle. Perform ten times clockwise and ten times counterclockwise. Perform with one eye at a time, and both eyes together.

Important Eye Note: Breathe deeply and naturally and try not to blink. See the letter as clearly as possible without eye strain. These Egyptian Eye Techniques are superior exercises for reshaping the eye-balls and strengthening the eye muscles. They help to create eye muscle balance. Do not confuse this exercise with ordinary eye exercises—there is no comparison!

The **Egyptian Letter Gazing Technique** enables the eyes to focus in all directions and allows both eyes to see together. It also helps to reshape the eye back to its normal position, so that light can focus on the retina properly for perfect eyesight. This technique coordinates the mind and eyes to work in perfect harmony. Practice will bring improvement. Stick with it! Persistence is the key to success in vision improvement.

Pre-school children naturally look in all directions with their eyes. School children are taught to look directly ahead and down at their books. After many years of this poor eye habit, they stop looking in all directions, and the eyeball loses its natural shape. Consequently, vision problems result.

Advanced Egyptian Letter Gazing Technique - Part II

After practicing the **Egyptian Letter Gazing Technique Part I**, with your card one foot in front of your eyes, for a month, you can now practice the **Advanced Egyptian Letter Gazing Technique, Part II.**

How to Perform: Hold the card at least two to three feet from your eyes. To improve the distant sight, you must use the eyes to see beyond two feet to overcome myopia (nearsightedness). Paste a black letter on a 2 by 3 card and tape the card to one end of a 12 inch ruler. These letters should be big enough for you to see easily at two foot. As your eyesight becomes clear at this distance, you can use smaller letters to help you obtain further improvement.

To improve your close vision (farsightedness), simply perform the eye exercise holding the letters less than twelve inches from your eyes. Perform this "Advanced" exercise in the same sequence as you did in the above Beginning Egyptian Letter Gazing Technique - Part I.

Important Note for Egyptian Letter Gazing Technique:
When working on your close vision, use a black letter that you can see clearly, but do not move it in to the point where you cannot see it clearly. The same goes for distant vision. Take your time in moving the card closer or further. For example, bring the card "in" one inch only every few weeks for close vision (far-sightedness), but be sure you can see the letters sharp and clear! The same holds true for distant vision (nearsightedness)—an inch or two at a time every few weeks. Don't be in a hurry to force your eyes to see better.

Perfect Eyesight

Eye Exercise Three
Yoga Accommodative Eye Exercise
(To Improve Close and Distant Vision)

The ancient Hindu Yogi's devised many techniques for improving the eyesight. This marvelous eye exercise helps the eyes to improve their ability to **change focus** and see clearly in the distance and at the close-point.

Modern science tells us that the "accommodative eye muscles" weaken with age. However, this is not true, if you continue to use the accommodative focusing eye muscles regularly, your eyesight will remain clear and strong throughout life. If you have lost this "accommodative eye focusing ability," this eye exercise can bring back your natural eye accommodation for distance and close-point seeing. This exercise mainly helps farsightedness or old age sight, the ability to focus at the close-point clearly.

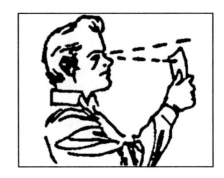

Figure 3-3

Practice the **Yoga Accommodative Exercise** outside in good light or inside in a well lighted room, while looking out the window. Here's how to perform the Hindu Yoga Accommodative Eye Exercise: **(Figure 3.3).**

Step One: Pick out a distant object, about twenty feet or more away (tree, car, building etc. This is your object; see it clearly. Now, move your eyes back to a letter on the card (at the close point) and see it clearly for a few seconds. Perform this accommodative eye movement three times (in and out).

Step Two: In your hand, hold a 2 x 3 card with black letters, and large enough for you to see clearly.

Step Three: Hold card at eye level, and at arm's length away, or where you can see it clearly.

Step Four: Look at a distant object, i.e., road sign, car, tree; see it clearly. Next, move your eyes back to a letter on the card (at the close point) and see it clearly or a few seconds. Perform 3 times or more, close-in and far-out—in and out.

Step Five: When the letter on the card becomes easier to see, then move the card a couple inches closer and repeat this "close point and distant point" movement three times, as in **Step Four**.

Step Six: Next, move the card a few inches closer, while still seeing it clearly. Again, repeat the "close" and "distant" eye movement, always focusing your eyes as clearly as you can.

Perfect Eyesight

Practice this Yoga Eye Exercise one eye at a time, then with both eyes together. Eventually, you'll be able to **see** the letters on the card at the close point, four or five inches from your eyes, clear and sharp.

The accommodative eye muscles, just like any other body muscles, become weaker, **not as a result of age, but of disuse.** Muscles are made to be exercised. The eyes are no different than body muscles. What works for one, physiologically, biologically and mechanically, will work for the other. If the eye muscles are strengthened, fresh blood begins to flow to them, and the eyes therefore become stronger, with improved vision.

Important Eye Muscle Note: When you perform arm, chest and back exercises with weights or machines regularly, your muscles grow strong. Eye exercises induce fresh blood flow, chi flow and nerve force to the eye muscles and nerves, thereby enhancing vision. This Special Yoga Exercise prevents the accommodative eye focusing muscles from weakening, and also to regain its elasticity. Perform this movement two or three times a week.

Eye Exercise Four
Yoga Accommodative Eye Exercise.
(To Improve Distant Vision)

Follow the steps in **Eye Exercise Three,** but reverse the procedure by looking at a card with letters on it, held at reading distance, 15 to 18 inches away from your eyes. Hold the card where you are able to see the 'letters' clearly, then immediately look at any object twenty feet away, i.e., tree, car, building etc. Next, focus your eyes from the card to the distant object, seeing both as clearly as possible, three times back and forth. Next, look at an object twenty to thirty feet further away than the first object. Repeat the back and forth eye movement three times. Continue with this exercise as you look at objects further into the distance. Practice this distance seeing accommodative eye movement for five minutes, two or three times a week.

Eye Exercise Five
Tai Chi Rocker Eye Technique--An Amazing Discovery
(To Improve Close and Distant Vision)

If all the time you have is five or ten minutes, the **Tai Chi Rocker Eye Technique** will give your eyes a thorough workout and strengthen your eye focusing muscles.

While studying and practicing Chi Kung and Tai Chi exercises, I made an amazing discovery—a new way to improve the eyesight with a Chi Kung movement called the **"Tai Chi Rocker"** Exercise, **Figure 4.3.** It is an invaluable eye exercise to improve both the close and distant vision.

Tai Chi Rocker relaxes the eyes, strengthens the focusing muscles, centers and grounds the mind, body and spirit. Practice this exercise for five to ten minutes, two or three times a week.

Place the small eye chart on the wall at eye level. (See **Chart 1** on page 34). Shine a bright light on the chart to prevent eye strain. Stand two or three feet away from the chart. Place your right foot six inches in front of the left. Gaze at one of the letters on the chart that you can see easily.

To start, begin to rock back and forth. When rocking backward the front right foot comes up and the back foot stays flat on the ground. While rocking forward the back of the left foot raises upward, while the front right foot stays on the ground. Rock back and forth for one or two minutes. Relax, and allow the letter on the chart to become clear in your vision. Distant vision improves by seeing the letter clearer as you move backward, Rock Forward, left heel up away from the chart, and Close vision improves. Rock back, right toe up as you move forward, toward the chart

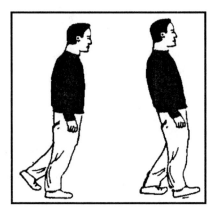

Figure 4.3
Rock forward, left heel up. Rock backward, right toe up.

Note: For close vision improvement only, rock within 2 feet of the chart; do not move further back. To improve your distant vision, you can move back as far as you can see the letters on the chart—five to sixty feet away.

Next, switch the position of your feet. Place your left foot forward and the right foot behind you. Practice the "rocking" movement for one to two minutes.

Every two to three minutes close your eyes and relax your body. Feel your eyes becoming softer and more relaxed. Also, remember the black "letter" clearly in your mind. For best results, close your eyes and place both palms over eyes for fifteen seconds (see **"palming technique"** Eye Exercise Nine).

Perfect Eyesight

Chart 1: Snellen Eye Chart Test Card

Fifty Feet.

A

Thirty Feet.

C G

Twenty Feet.

F E P

Fifteen Feet.

L Z O D

Ten Feet.

C N G A B

Five Feet.

H A Q O E

Three Feet.

Z U K L T P A

Two Feet.

B R O C G D N

Perfect Eyesi

Vital Points to Remember While Performing The Tai Chi Rocker Technique

Point 1: To improve close vision, rock toward the chart and stop rocking forward as soon as the letter on the chart starts to blur, then rock back.

Point 2: To improve distant vision, move further away from the chart. Imagine "pulling" the letters out of the eye chart as you rock backward. As you rock forward, notice the "letter" becoming more clear.

Point 3: Remember to perform the "Palming Technique" every two minutes; try to soften and relax your eyes and mind.

Point 4: Shine a bright light on the eye chart to prevent eye strain. Or perform the eye exercises in the outdoor natural light.

Point 5: Focus on the eye chart letters with a soft, relaxed look.

Point 6: Never hold your breath. Breathe deeply and gently.

Point 7: Practice with one eye at a time. Place palm over one eye while both eyes are open--this enables both eyes to work together. Finally, practice with both eyes together.

Perform Yoga stretching movements after performing the **Tai Chi Rocker Eye Technique.** Reach for the sky with both hands and one hand at a time, bend over and touch your toes; stretch backward, to the sides; roll your neck in circles. Stretching releases tension, improves blood and nerve circulation to the eyes. (See chapter on Chi Kung Stretching Exercises).

Eye Exercise Six
Close Vision Strengthening Exercises

Close Vision Technique A:
(Accommodative "Whipping Eye Technique")

"Whipping' is one of the best eye exercises for strengthening the accommodative eye muscles to **improve close vision.**

How to perform the Whipping Eye Exercise: Cup your left palm over your left eye. Hold a card with a black letter on it, that you can easily see, at arms' length in front of your eyes. Pull the card toward your right eye at a moderate speed within a few inches of your face. Next, quickly 'whip' the card suddenly back to arm's length. Repeat this movement several times. Then, use the left eye while the right eye is cupped with your right palm. Repeat several times. Next, practice 'whipping' with both eyes open at the same time. Repeat several times. Perform two to three times a week. "Whipping" is an exercise that greatly helps presbyopia (middle-age sight), Farsightedness, and any other close vision problems.

Close Vision Technique B:
"Tromboning"

How to Perform the Tromboning Eye Exercise: Hold out a card, with a small black letter you can easily see at arms' length. From arms length, 'slide' (move) the card three inches toward your right eye, then move it back to arms' length. Next, 'slide' the card six inches toward your right eye, then move it back out to arms length. Next, 'slide' the card nine inches toward your right eye, then move it back out to arms length. Progress in this manner three inches at a time until the card is a couple inches away from your eye. Practice several times with your right eye. Next, perform "Tromboning" with your left eye, then with both eyes together.

Move the card at a moderate easy speed. Relax and breathe easily. After practicing this exercise for a few weeks, vary the speed of the card—moving the card more slowly, other times at a brisk speed. Consistently practiced, Whipping and Tromboning eventually awakens and strengthens the focusing muscles for the close point, to where you can see the print sharp and clear.

Close Vision Technique C:
"Close Point Eye Sharpening Technique"

Many people go through middle age with blurry vision at the close point. This does not have to happen. You can do something about it. And this exercise, as well as the previous one is a positive step in doing something to strengthen and improve your close vision.

I have found this "Close Point Eye Sharpening Technique," when performed correctly, to be the most important eye technique to improve close vision. It is easy to do and only needs to be practiced twice a week. This is the latest eye improvement technique that I devised in 1995. **(Figure 4-4)** below. Here's how it's done: (See "Principles of Eye Training Chart" Page 38).

Step 1: Hold **"Principles of Eye Training Chart"** in front of your eyes, from 12 to 20 inches, where you can see it without strain.

Step 2: Trace the first letter of the first (1.) paragraph with your eyes, for example, "V" in "Vision."

Step 3. Close your eyes and trace and visualize the letter "V" in your mind.

Perfect Eyesight

Step 4: Open your eyes, look at the letter "V" and trace it again.

Step 5: Close your eyes and trace letter "V" again, then open eyes while inhaling and exhaling a gentle deep breath, and look at the letter "V".

Step 6: Move the letter "V" "in" slowly towards your eyes while trying to see the letter as clearly as possible--when the letter starts to blur, stop the movement.

Step 7: Close your eyes for a few seconds. Open your eyes with a deep breath and move letter "V" away from your eyes, and notice the letter become clearer.

Step 8: Place both palms over eyes for twenty seconds, while visualizing a black color.

Repeat **Steps One through Eight** with the first letter of all eleven paragraphs on page 39, for example, "T" for paragraph #2, "R" for paragraph #3 and so forth. Or go down to the smallest paragraph that you can **see clearly.** Practice this exercise at least 15 to 20 minutes, two or three times a week.

**Move print card in and out
Follow Step 1 to Step 8**

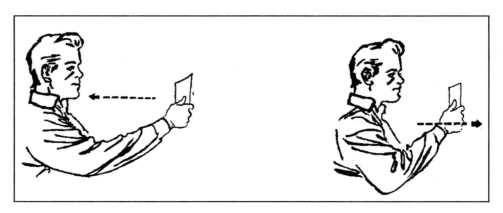

**Figure 4-4. Close Vision Technique C
"Close Point Eye Sharpening Technique"**

Perfect Eyesight

Close Vision – Chart 2
Principles of Eye Training Chart

1. Vision can be improved by natural methods.

2. Tension causes eye strain and impairs vision. Relaxation relieves tension.

3. Relaxed eyes are normal eyes. When eyes lose their relaxation and become tense, they strain and stare and the vision becomes poor.

4. Vision can be improved only by education in proper seeing. Proper seeing is relaxed seeing. Normal eyes shift rapidly and continuously. Eyes with defective vision become fixed and staring. When staring eyes learn to shift, vision improves.

5. The eyeball is like the camera, and changes in focal length. To focus the camera, you must adjust the distance from the negative to the front of the camera.

6. To focus the eye, the distance between the retina at the back ands the cornea in front must be increased for close vision and decreased for the distant view.

7. Six muscles on the outside of the eyeball control its shape; four, reaching from front to back, flatten the eye; two, belting it around the middle, squeeze it long from front to back.

8. When the eyes are relaxed, these six muscles are flexible and cooperate automatically, adjusting the focal length so eyes may see both near and far.

9. Just as dependence on crutches weakens leg muscles, so dependence on glasses weakens eye muscles by relieving them of responsibility. But muscles can be reeducated to do their duties.

10. Relaxation of the eyes and mind brings relaxation of the entire body. This general relaxation increases circulation and brings improved physical, visual and mental health.

11. Relaxation is a sensation.

Eye Exercise Seven
Stretch Your Vision
Distant Vision Strengthening Exercise
(To Improve Nearsightedness--Myopia)

This exercise was taught in Michigan, in the 1940s, by two optometrists, Drs. Ross and Rhymer. **"Stretch Your Vision"** is extremely valuable in extending the limits of your distant vision, especially for myopic vision (nearsightedness). **(Figures 5-3 and 6-3).**

Practice **"Stretch Your Vision"** at least 15 to 30 minutes, two or three times a week.

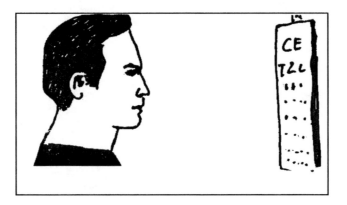

1) Look at Chart and trace letter.   2) Close eyes, relax body
3) Open eyes and look at letter.
Figure 5-3

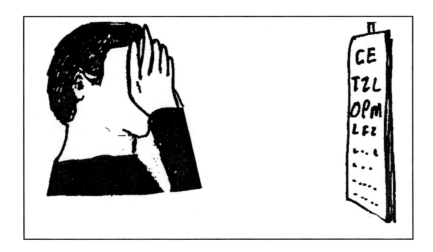

Palm 20 seconds. Open eyes with deep breath.
Look at letter and walk backwards
Figure 6-3

Perfect Eyesight

How to Perform the "Stretch Your Vision" Exercise: To start, place the Snellen Eye Chart 1 on page 30, on a wall at eye level. (See **Figure 5-3** and **6-3**)

Step 1: Stand straight and select one of the "letters" on the chart.

Step 2: Trace your chosen "letter" in your mind, then close your eyes for a few seconds. Relax your hands, shoulders, eyes, legs, neck etc.

Step 3: Open your eyes and look at the letter again. Next, place both palms over eyes and "Palm" while visualizing the "letter" in your mind for 15 seconds.

Step 4: Open your eyes with a deep inhalation and exhalation of breath, noticing the "letter" becoming blacker.

Step 5: While looking at the "letter", begin swaying slowly from side to side. While you continue to sway, move s-l-o-w-l-y away from the chart, taking very short backward steps. Breathe naturally and allow the print to come in clearly. When you reach the point where the print becomes indistinct or unreadable, STOP! At this point, bend forward at the waist, continuing to sway, and again read the "letter". Now, resume your short backward steps.

Again, even though learning far forward, you will reach the point at which the printed letters are no longer legible. When this occurs, straighten up, move close to the chart and repeat the exercise on the next smaller line, following the above instructions. Repeat each line until you reach the bottom line of the chart.

It is important to relax the entire body while performing this exercise. Mentally and physically feel your shoulders, neck, face, eye, arms and hands relax. Let go of your jaw muscles and let them drop. Let your eyes become soft and calm.

<u>Important Note on Lighting</u>: **When performing this exercise inside, be sure a bright light shines on your Snellen Eye Chart to prevent eye strain. Perform "Stretch Your Vision" two or three times a week. Use a 150 to 200 watt bulb or a bright flood light on the Chart.**

Stick To It . . . You Must Give It Time!

Perfect Eyesight

Eye Exercise Eight
Test Card Eye Exercise
(To Improve Close and Distant Vision)

Dr. Bates recommended this eye exercise to help strengthen ones' distant and close vision. It can be performed during your regular routine, or during spare moments throughout the day. It is also a great eye exercise for those who have already achieved good eyesight, and want to maintain their excellent vision.

Stand two feet away from the **Snellen Eye Chart 1,** page 34:

Step 1: Look at the top Eye Chart Letter 'A'—trace it with your eyes or nose.

Step 2: Close eyes for five seconds. Relax eyes and open with a gentle breath, and notice the letter 'A' looking blacker and clearer.

Step 3: Palm eyes for twenty seconds. Open eyes with a gentle breathe, and notice the letter blacker and clearer.

Step 4: Look at the next line 'C' 'G' on the Eye Chart. Repeat the above sequence.

Perform these Four Steps all the way down to the bottom line on the Eye Chart. When you can see the bottom line, move three inches closer to the Eye Chart. Each week move closer, but do not be in any hurry to do this if you cannot see the Eye Chart letters clearly. In other words, move 'closer' ONLY when the letters come in clearly. Never strain to see the Eye Chart. Persistent and dedicated practice with this exercise

However, you can move closer to the Eye Chart when working with the upper, larger letter-lines even if you cannot see the lower smaller lines. Move closer to the upper larger lines that you can see clearly. The goal is to read the smallest line at four or five inches away. If you can do this, you'll have perfect eyesight at the close point. Practice two or three times weekly, until you achieve this goal.

Perfect Eyesight

Distant Vision Exercise
Stand three feet away from the **Snellen Eye Chart 1.**

Step 1: Look at letter 'A' at the top of the Eye Chart—now trace letter 'A'

Step 2: Close your eyes for five seconds. Next, open your eyes with a gentle breath, and notice the letter 'A' gets blacker and clearer.

Step 3: Palm your eyes for twenty seconds. Next, open eyes with a gentle breath, and notice the 'A' blacker and clearer.

Step 4: Look at the next line 'C' 'G' on the Eye Chart. Repeat the above sequence.

Perform the **Four Steps** all the way down to the bottom line on the **Snellen Eye Chart.** When you can see the bottom line, move one foot further away from the Eye Chart. Each week move farther back, but do not be in any hurry to do this if you cannot see the Eye Chart letters clearly. In other words, move further back **only** when the letters come in clearly. Never strain to see the Letters on the Eye Chart.

However, you can move further back when working with the top five lines on the Eye Chart, even if you cannot see the lower smaller lines. Move further back on the upper larger letter-lines you can see clearly.

Eye Exercise Nine
Tibetan Peripheral Vision Technique

How important is peripheral vision? Everyone uses their peripheral vision while driving, walking, playing sports, at work and at home. In fact, if we didn't use our peripheral vision, we would develop "tunnel vision," just like the old gray mare going down the street with blinders attached to the sides of his eyes. He can only look forward. He is blind to everything around him.

We develop "tunnel vision" or lack of peripheral vision by concentrating to "hard" with the eyes fixed forward. We concentrate in a 'fixed hard gaze', straight in front of us, and we lose the ability to see clearly peripherally (side-vision).

How well do you see on the sides? Before being taught to read, children can see with their side (peripheral) vision clear and sharp. The great sports athletes like Wayne Gretsky, Barry Sanders and Michael Jordan are praised by their peers for having "eyes behind their head." They have developed extremely good peripheral vision. They know where the ball or puck is at every moment.

With strong, well-developed side vision, you can prevent accidents while driving your car. Your ability to play any sport will improve dramatically. Dr. William H. Bates, the

Perfect Eyesight

famous eye specialist says, **"The normal eye sees one thing BEST, but not one thing only."** By developing your "Peripheral" (side vision), you too can have "eyes behind your head."

Your eyes must be gazing straight forward, without movement to either side. Just pay attention to what is going on "peripherally," on your right and left.

How to perform the "Tibetan Peripheral Vision Technique":

Step 1: Hold a pencil in each hand, twelve inches in front of your eyes. **Figure 7-3.**

Step 2: Gaze straight out past the pencils into the "distance", without looking directly at the pencils. See the pencils with your "Peripheral Vision." **Do not** look directly at the pencils.

Step 3: Move each pencil s-l-o-w-l-y to the sides of each eye, as far as you can see them peripherally. Repeat this front-to-side movement at least ten times.

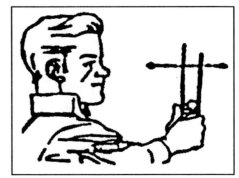

Figure 7-3

Step 4: Next, move the pencils, right hand upward and left hand downward, ten times.

Step 5: Next, move the pencils right hand diagonally upward, and left hand diagonally downward, ten times.

Step 6: Next, move the pencils left hand diagonally upward, and right hand diagonally downward, ten times.

Step 7: Next, hold pencils twelve inches in front of your eyes and make a circle about two or three feet in diameter, from the center of head out to the sides. Keep your eyes looking straight ahead in all seven Steps. Perform circles clockwise and counterclockwise.

Important Eye Training Note: Allow your side vision to come into focus "naturally" without effort. Do not strain to "see" peripherally. When you walk, drive or read, use your peripheral vision to see the buildings, cars, furniture and people around you. Blocking-out the side vision creates eye muscle imbalance and is a major cause of imperfect eyesight. Many accidents can be prevented with well-developed peripheral vision. Practice the Peripheral Vision Technique three to five minutes, two to three times a week.

Perfect Eyesight

Eye Exercise Ten
Dr. Bates' and Yoga Eye Palming Techniques
(Always finish eye exercises with palming)

Palming was re-discovered by William H. Bates, M.D. in the early 1900s. The ancient Indian Yogis and Chinese Taoists practiced eye palming techniques for thousands of years. They "palmed" their eyes as a form of meditation or inner visualization and relaxation. "Palming" is performed by gently 'cupping' both palms over the eyes, blocking out as much light as possible. Palm for five minutes daily. The Masters say that too much outward gazing at all the 'exciting', bright and fast-moving things in the world upsets the inner balance of our 'spiritual third eye. Our physical eyes and brain become clouded, confused and agitated, like a muddy stream. Palming calms our mind, emotions, spirit and body. Our inner and outer eyes take on the qualities of a clear, tranquil, peaceful pool of water. When our mind is tranquil, our eyesight focuses on the world with clarity and insight.

Palming is one of the most important methods for relaxing eye muscles, eye nerves. Palming helps to calm the mind; improve color clarity; and is very helpful for many degenerative eye conditions when performed regularly.

Palming Soothes and Rests the Eyes

Palming is practiced and taught by many Visual Training Teachers throughout the world, i.e., Germany, the Yogis of India, Chinese Taoists, Tibetan Monks, Naturopaths, and Holistic Doctors everywhere.

This superior technique can bring about a complete transformation and restoration of your eyes. When you learn how to palm correctly, you'll be inspired to palm daily, because it relaxes the eyes, the body and the mind.

When you first start palming, you may see gray, white light or colors. As you continue practicing, however, you will see only black darkness. You have reached a state of calm, your mind is relaxed and your eyes can heal and regenerate quickly.

"Let Go" Mentally While Palming

While palming, "let go" mentally, because your eyes cannot completely relax when the mind or body is full of stress and tension. The brain is like a camera—we see through the brain. You can strain the eyes while palming, if your brain is in "tension," thinking about your problems, the same as you can with them open. You must relax your "brain-stuff" (thoughts) while palming. Then you will "see" improved eyesight. For complete relaxation, breathe slowly, evenly and naturally. Give your problems to the Universe or Higher Power. Let your mind dwell on something beautiful-a blue ocean, sandy beach, sunset, mountains, a loving face etc.

Complete relaxation leads to complete healing this is your goal! Avoid strain or force while palming. Shut out all light and think of a black box lined with black velvet. When your inner mind is able to see, visualize and remember BLACK while palming, your vision will improve.

How to Perform the Yoga Fetal Palming Technique

The Yogis of India discovered that performing palming in the Fetal Kneeling Position or Fetal Squatting Position is more relaxing and healing than in the upright sitting position. However, all three palming positions are beneficial and can be performed at any time.

Always finish your eye exercise routine with palming. Palming in the kneeling or squatting position is an excellent method of complete eye, mind, and body relaxation. Fresh blood circulation and nerve flow to the eyes are also greatly enhanced.

Kneeling Fetal Position
Palming Technique: Figure 8-3.
While kneeling in the fetal position (on knees and body bent forward, face down), bring head to floor in front of knees, with "cupped" palms over eyes). Rest the heel of your palms on your cheek bones, fingers crossed over your forehead. Be sure your palms do not touch the eyeballs; keep out as much light as possible. Visualize BLACK VELVET.

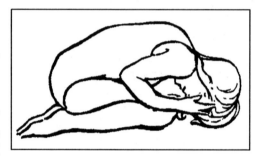

Figure 8-3

Squatting Fetal Position Palming Technique: Squat down with feet eight to ten inches apart. Place arms over your knees and cup palms over eyes. Relax in this position with palms covering eyes. In the East people squat in this position to have babies, eat and eliminate. It is a natural position and very conducive to relaxation, meditation and palming.

Important Eye Improvement Note:
When you palm correctly, you will see "perfect blackness." The blacker you see while palming, the faster your eyesight improves. Perfect blackness equals perfect eyesight. Perfect blackness indicates that your visual nerve senses are relaxed and are functioning correctly.

If you see gray or various colors while palming, it indicates that your vision is unclear and blurry. Palming while visualizing "black" helps to darken the palm area. You cannot "force" blackness in the "palming field area." Mentally forcing to "see" black, creates more tension and weak vision. To see perfect blackness, visualize anything black, i.e., black cat, dog, car, shoes etc. Relax mind, body and spirit and let blackness come in.

Perfect Eyesight

After each eye exercise session, palm for at least **five minutes**. Relax! After palming, open your eyes and notice how the trees, grass, sky, houses, people appear clear, bright and more colorful.

Heal Liver and Eyes with the Color of Green

In the Orient, the Taoist Masters teach us that "green" is associated with the liver and the eyes. Green vegetables and nature's green colors—trees, grass etc., help to heal the liver and also heal your eyes too! Gently visualize green trees, green grass, blue-green ocean, and your eyes and mind become calmer, happier and more peaceful. You can palm at any time you feel the need to relax and let go—it refreshes your mind and rejuvenates your eyes.

The Sit Down Palming Technique

Place palms over your eyes, elbows on table, with back and neck straight. You can use a small pillow under your elbows if you wish; this helps to relax your arms. Use this method at work if you are unable to perform the Fetal Floor Palming Technique. (You wouldn't want to be caught on the floor when your boss walks in)! Both palming techniques will work. Just "do it" and "see" your vision improve. Happy Palming!

The Secret 'Black Globe' Palming Technique

The real inner secret behind perfect eyesight is to **relax the eyes, body, brain and mind completely**! Complete relaxation means complete healing of body, mind and vision. To do this, you must be able to visualize totally black space while palming with your eyes closed.

When you think that you have pictured, while palming, a background as black as it can be, imagine a "round" very black "Globe" pictured against that back-ground. What do you see? You will see something still blacker than that background. Then let go of the background and let the Black Globe spread out until it becomes the background itself.

Try to picture a still blacker Globe on the new background and so on, until you get a background so black that nothing blacker can be imagined. Perfect blackness equals perfect relaxation, and perfect relaxation equals perfect vision.

Ten to fifteen minutes of "seeing black" while palming will prove to you what a marvelous relaxation technique this is. Some people have reported eye strain relieved in only a few palming sessions. After "seeing black", you will be able to see much more clearly and strongly—either at the close point or far point. To see the fullest degree of "blackness", first look at a perfectly black object, i.e., black car, black cat/dog, black velvet etc., and then (while palming) try to **remember** that blackness.

The Key to Seeing Perfect Blackness

Perfect blackness that is recalled and perceived, indicates that the mind is perfectly relaxed. When you cultivate the power to "remember black," your brain/mind is relaxed and rested, instantaneously, and your eyesight strengthened tremendously.

Your mastery in remembering to see black goes beyond relaxation. It enables you to see much "blacker" the letters on a page, thus making them sharper and easier to read. Practice a few minutes each day and you will see marked improvement. Your subconscious memory of "perfect blackness", carried in your mind when your eyes are open, will give you a high degree of mental and visual clarity and strength. Thus, your vision can be improved immediately, if your memory and mental image of "perfect blackness" is visualized and retained.

For best results in eye improvement, practice Palming every single day. If you "make time" for your Palming Exercise, time will be good to your eyes in your golden years.

Bates and other natural eye training specialists state that many cases of imperfect eyesight—nearsightedness, farsightedness, aging vision—have been permanently cured by the simple practice of "seeing black" while palming over a period of time.

The Amazing Master Formulas Behind "Perfect Eyesight"

It has been discovered in ancient writings from ages past that the brain/mind and the eyes operate in close harmony. Defective eyesight can be improved by mental methods accompanied by proper eye habits, eye exercises, diet and physical relaxation techniques.

This amazing "secret" to Perfect Eyesight lies in the coordination between the brain and the muscles controlling the movements of the eyeball.

The Three Master Formulas to Perfect Eyesight
Master Eye Formula Number One
Relax the Eye Muscles

Abnormal strain of the external muscles of the eyes is always associated by a strained, unnatural effort to see. When this strain is stopped, the eye muscles become normal and all errors of refraction vanish like magic. In each "error of refraction" there is a different kind of strain. Relaxing any type of eye strain will relieve that particular error of refraction. In other words, total relaxation of eye, mind and body reduces all "errors of refraction." When one is angry, stressed-out or tense, vision becomes blurry. Relaxation brings clarity. **Master Eye Formula Technique One:** Palm and visualize absolute black, while breathing-in healing light into your eyes, hold for a second, and breathe-out through the bottom of your feet. Perform 10 or 20 breaths daily.

Master Eye Formula Number Two
Relax the Brain and Mind

Eye tension or strain to see is literally a strain and tension of your mind; conversely, when your mind strains, it is reflected as a strain of the eyes. Therefore, we see a very true connection between stressed-out mental states and defective eyesight, each acting upon and reacting to the other in a cause and effect relationship. **Master Eye Formula Technique Two:** Sit, relax mind, and visualize a peaceful sunset or sunrise. Breathe-in energy going up the back of your spine; next, exhale, visualizing chi-energy going down front of your body, and inhale back up the spine. This relaxes any tension in your body, mind or spirit, and allows vision to come naturally. Perform 10 or 20 times daily.

Master Eye Formula Number Three
Reduce Mental Strain and Strengthen Eye Muscles

The only real treatment for regaining your lost eyesight begins by relieving mental stress and strain, followed by a recovery of the mental control of the eye muscles. The vision exercises in this book will help you reduce mental strain, physical stress and allow your eye muscles to strengthen and function in a relaxed manner, as they were meant to do **Master Eye Formula Technique Three:** Lie down, place both palms over lower abdomen, tongue near roof of month, but not touching. Next, breath-in, push-out lower abdomen, and visualize golden healing light coming into your abdomen. Exhale, and your belly goes back down. Repeat 10 or 20 times daily, upon arising and at bed-time. It helps you to sleep soundly by taking "thinking energy" out of your head, and places it in the healing hara-belly center of your body. This technique reduces mental stress, and helps heal your entire body, mind and eyes.

Important Eye Note: Dr. Bates once said:
"When the mind is at rest, nothing can tire the eyes; and
when the mind is under a strain nothing can rest them;
anything that rests the mind will benefit the eyes."

Do you want Perfect Eyesight? Develop mental poise and balance—a prerequisite of mental relaxation and removal of strain. Learn to "let go" of mental strain, worry, fear, anxiety, etc. Practice mental calm and watch your eyesight improve by quantum leaps!

Important Inspirational Eye Training Note:
Your eyes are your most precious possession. Consistent practice of the eye techniques in this chapter will allow you to always keep your eyesight clear and sharp for a long, healthy and happy lifetime. Stick with it! You must give your eyes time to strengthen and heal. Let it be done! We wish you much success in your quest for "Perfect Eyesight."

What is Progressive Eye Training?

Each month make your eye routine more progressive and challenging. Perform more repetitions. Walk back further away from the eye chart. Increase Palming time and frequency. Change your eye routine or perform different eye exercise for your specific eye condition.

Progressive eye training exercises increase circulation to the eyes for quicker eye improvement. If your eyes get overly sore or fatigued from eye training, take a rest-break for a couple days from your eye routine to allow nerve, tendon and eye muscle healing and repair.

Always move your eyes smoothly during your eye muscle exercises. Smooth eye movements relax the eyes, which helps you to see clearly. Keep practicing until you perform all eye routines smoothly and calmly. When you reach Perfect Eyesight—20-10 or better, a 15 minute eye routine, once a week, is enough to maintain perfect vision. Also, continue your daily natural eye habits for life. You can prevent eye problems and maintain Perfect Eyesight for as long as you live. Be Healthy and Prosper!

Eyesight Training Exercise Schedule
Weekly Eye Training Program

1. Eye Muscle Exercises - 5 to 10 minutes two or three times a week.
2. Side Vision Exercises (Peripheral) - 5 minutes, two or three times a week.
3. Distance Seeing Exercises (Nearsighted) - 15 to 30 minutes, 2-3 times a week.
4. Close Seeing Exercises (Farsighted) - 15 to 30 minutes, 2-3 times a week.
5. Yoga Neck Rolls - 3 minutes, two or three times a week. Head, Face, Eye Massage - 5 minutes, two or three times a week.
6. Taoist Internal Chi Kung Exercises-15 minutes, 2-3 times a week. See Chapter Four.

Daily Eye and Health Enhancement Program

1. Eye Palming - 5 to 10 minutes Daily.
2. Eye or Nose Edging and Tracing (Close & Distant) 3 to 5 minutes.
3. Practice distance seeing throughout the day.
4. Look up from your close work every 10-15 minutes.
5. Hold book or reading material at Least 20 Inches from Eyes.
6. Sit and stand with good posture.
7. Eat wholesome and nutritious foods for your body type.
8. Stop eating lifeless junk food.
9. Obtain sufficient rest and sleep.
10. Go outside daily in the fresh air and sunshine.
11. Go outside or take a slow walk after eating.
12. Use natural, whole-food vitamins, minerals and herbs daily.
13. Use herbal eye drops or take an herbal eye bath with "eye cup."
14. Head Lift Technique.

Chapter Four

Internal Chi Kung Energy Exercises for Vision Improvement

How to Build a Strong Healthy Constitution

Good posture and internal organ health is vitally important for clear sharp vision. The Yogis and Chi Kung Masters practice stretching and posture exercises to strengthen their kidneys and lower back area. The kidneys are considered the health and longevity organs of the body. If you want to stay young, vibrant and full of energy, practice these internal exercises daily. See **Figure 1-4,** next page.

These powerful exercise movements have been taught and practiced throughout the world in every culture to improve health, increase longevity, enhance vision and spiritual clarity. These are important energy exercises for you to perform daily for the rest of your life. Make these movements a daily habit, and you'll be rewarded by great health and vitality.

Internal Exercise Number One
Kidney and Lower Back Strengthening Movement

Chinese Traditional Doctors say that the kidneys are the Mother Organs of the body. They regulate water and protein in the body. Too much or not enough of each can result in poor health and illness. Kidneys are considered our constitutional longevity organ. Strong kidneys impart calmness to the mind and spirit. Weak kidneys instill fear and trembling throughout the body, mind and spirit. This Kidney Exercise will help to strengthen your kidneys and lower back **Figure 1-4**.

How to perform the Kidney and Lower Back Exercise: Figure 1-4. First, stand with feet close together. Reach forward, without bending the knees; look upward with your eyes and bend forward while trying to touch the floor with your hands. Feel the stretch in your lower back. Looking up keeps your back straight. This movement normalizes the lower back, strengthens the kidneys and helps you to stay grounded and balanced. Perform six times.

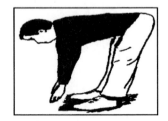

Figure 1-4

Internal Exercise Number Two
Spine Straightening Movement

Good posture is the key to good energy-chi circulation to the eyes and body organs that feed nourishment to the eyes. This simple exercise is invaluable for improving and maintaining a healthy, strong posture for life.

How to Perform the "Spine Straightening Movement": Simply, let your head fall backward while standing in an upright posture. Hold this position for 15 seconds. This simple movement straightens the spine and raises the chest. Your body becomes gracefully poised, with a straight posture. Perform this movement several times a day. This posture enables your lungs to expand and breathe more deeply; it makes it easier for the blood to circulate through the heart and imparts more confidence.

Internal Exercise Number Three
Reaching for Heaven

This movement also benefits the eyesight, ears, complexion; increases lung capacity and respiration; stimulates the liver, kidneys, stomach, intestines and colon; helps to overcome constipation, improves sex gland function, trims, tones and strengthens and flattens the abdomen; overcomes fatigue and increases energy. Stretch up to the sky and watch your energy zoom!

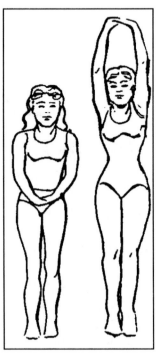

Figure 2-4

Perfect Eyesight

How to Perform "Reaching for Heaven": Figure 2-4. (Previous Page).

Stand with your feet 12 inches apart, with arms in front of body and fingers intertwined. Inhale a gentle deep breath while lifting your arms up above your head and stretching up on your toes. You can keep your head forward, or for variation, look upward at your hands. Then, hold your breath and stretch your arms upward and hold for a few seconds. Exhale, lower your arms down sideways. This movement helps to remove the 'hump' out of the upper back and straightens the spine and posture. This natural upward stretch breaks-up the blockages in the body for improved circulation and greater health. Repeat six times.

Internal Exercise Number Four
Tibetan Rejuvenation Rite

The Tibetan Rejuvenation Rite comes from the Tibetan Monks high up in the Himalayan Mountains in northern India. This powerful 'Rite" builds in the following ways: Strengthens the back and shoulder muscles; neck and leg areas; increases blood and nerve circulation to the brain and vital internal organs; helps to overcome constipation, slows down the aging process; increases lung capacity and breathing ability; overcomes lung problems; trims, tones and firms the waist and buttocks; helps bring circulation, blood and nerve force healing to the eyes.

How to Perform the Tibetan Rejuvenation Rite: Figure 3-4.

Lie on your stomach and place hands on the floor, shoulder width apart. Next, push upper body (shoulders and head) up and back, with hips almost touching floor—stretch neck and upper body as far back as possible. From this position raise on toes and hands, while lifting your hips straight up, while pointing the top of your head to the floor and touching your chin to your chest. Breathe "in" as your hips are raised, and breathe "out" when raising your head. Start with 6 repetitions and work up to 15 or 20. You'll feel invigorated and full of chi energy!

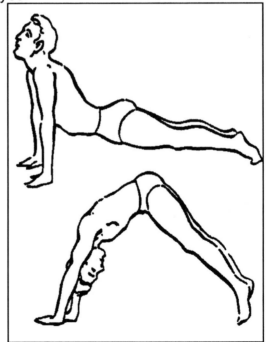

Figure 3-4

Perfect Eyesight

Internal Exercise Number Five
Sufi Bear Walk (Egyptian)

Perform this "walk" for one minute for a month, and add one minute each month until you are walking on all fours for three minutes. **Figure 4-4.** The Sufi Bear Walk strengthens the nerves and allows fresh blood to circulate directly to the eyes and brain. It tones the shoulder, back, arm and leg muscles. When you "walk" fast, you'll increase your endurance and stamina. Bears have a straight and powerful posture. It rebuilds postural muscles and overcomes the downward gravitational pull, which helps to overcome falling organs. It also imparts an internal massage to the abdomen and colon, thus helping to alleviate constipation and gastrointestinal problems. Perform at least three times per week.

**How to Perform the "Sufi Bear Walk":
Figure 4-4.**
Babies and animals walk on all four limbs in a 'cross-crawl' fashion like a bear, dog or cat. This exercise takes some practice to perform correctly. You have to bring your opposite arm and leg forward while moving forward on all fours, just like a bear. Using opposite arms and legs on all fours activates the right and left hemispheres of the brain, bringing balance and harmony to the body/mind connection.

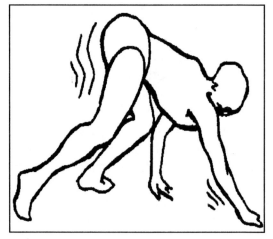

Figure 4-4

Internal Exercise Number Six
Jade Hop

This is a powerful "grounding" exercise. Too much thinking, worrying, reading, computers and other close work cause our energy to stay in our head-- we become ungrounded and unstable. We become top heavy and not centered in the Hara, which is two inches below the belly button. Life becomes difficult when we have excessive energy in the thinking head-brain. However, when we learn to ground our energy in our Hara-Ab area, answers to our problems come more easily; we see life as it is. When we are grounded we feel more relaxed and calm to handle any situation life brings to us.

How to Perform the "Jade Hop": Stand and simply start hopping up and down, one or two inches, in a relaxed manner. Continue until you feel slightly winded, one or two minutes. This simple but potent exercise strengthens the sexual organs, stimulates the pituitary gland in the mid-brain and the thymus gland over the heart. It builds strength in the legs, rejuvenates the kidneys and adrenal glands. It also helps to prevent the formation of kidney stones. "The Jade Hop" de-congests the head, sinuses and lungs to allow fresh blood to circulate in the head and eyes for better vision. It's also helps to move and circulate the lymphatic system to detoxify the body and build immunity. You can also use a jump rope for variety.

Internal Exercise Number Seven
Centering Movement

After "Grounding,'" your energy moves into your legs and feet and away from your head, Centering your energy is next. When Grounded, the tough times of life are easier to handle. Centering your body places you in harmony with life to able to see the correct answer to your problems. This wonderful movement loosens the back and squeezes the internal organs.

How to Perform the "Centering Movement": Stand with your feet shoulder width apart and relax. Bend your knees slightly; let your arms hang loosely like ropes, while your mid-body and shoulders move. Let your breathing be natural. Move your right shoulder forward and up in a circle, and then lower it backward. Do the same with the left shoulder, moving it forward, up in a circle and back. As your left shoulder is moving upward and back, let your right shoulder come forward and up again. Alternate in this manner while twisting your waist with the rotating movement. Do not tighten-up while performing this exercise: YOU MUST RELAX! Become like a "rag-doll." Just hang loose!

When first starting this movement, perform easy, small shoulder and twisting movements; gradually increase to larger circles. Put a smile on your face and pretend you are doing a dance.

The "Centering Movement" helps to expel toxins from the body, absorbs fresh chi-energy, increases your vitality and heals the internal organs. While twisting and squeezing your internal organs, it massages them thoroughly; it helps to release gas, belching and rumbling sounds a sign of toxins being expelled from the body. It is also great for weight reduction, eases shoulder and back pain, and strengthens the sexual organs. It helps to drain and massage the lymphatic glands. At first, perform 16 times. Eventually, perform for three minutes non-stop.

Chapter Five

Special Oriental Dao-Yin: Self-Healing Massage Techniques for Healthy Eyesight

Vision Health and Healing Secrets

From the Orient has come stories of miraculous healing powers never before seen in the West. What do the Orientals' know that the West has yet to learn? One of their great secrets is a self-massage practice called Dao-Yin. The Chinese refer to self-massage practice as self-acupressure or working the meridian pressure points for the internal organs. Many of the Japanese and Chinese Sages who practice and teach Dao-Yin or Doe-In in Japan are reported to be well over 100 years young and going strong!

Along with Dao-Yin and Chi Kung Yoga self-cultivation practices, they consume mainly whole natural foods, consisting of whole vegetables, fruits, seeds, grains, herb tablets and herbal teas. By practicing these methods, they say, one's health, immune system and energy levels improve by quantum leaps.

All these health and energy cultivation exercises, in addition to wholesome nutrition, herbs, meditation and prayer, are the keys that have been taught by the ancient teachers of all religions to maintain super health and overcome illness. A dear friend of ours from Toronto, Frances B. was suffering from partial paralysis of her left arm. A few days of performing Dao-Yin and Chi Kung exercises, and she was able to move her arm freely and without any pain.

Dao-Yin has many varied techniques and modalities for self-healing. When you improve circulation to one part of the body, the healing benefits are felt in other parts of the body also. The following is a very simple Dao-Yin routine. Just simply "rub" and "massage" the following areas in this order:

Daily Oriental Dao-Yin Self-Healing Massage Routine

☯ Rub the crown of the head and temples for mental clarity.
☯ Rub the ears to heat-up the body and invigorate the kidneys.
☯ Rub the eyes to regenerate the liver, improve vision, and refresh the spirit.
☯ Rub the nose to help heal heart problems.
☯ Rub the mouth to help improve stomach digestion.
☯ Rub the nostrils and cheeks to eliminate mucus, sinus problems and to cleanse the lungs.
☯ Rub the neck for emotional problems, stress, and to increase vitality; also helps for calmness and poise.
☯ Rub the arms for heart problems, nervousness and emotional love problems.
☯ Rub the chest and upper back for depression, grief and the courage to face life without fear.
☯ Rub the heart area for greater circulation and spiritual love.
☯ Rub the liver (under right rib cage), to strengthen the eyesight and for sustaining energy.
☯ Rub the kidneys for better hearing or ear problems.
☯ Rub the big toe to clear the brain and achieve mental clarity.
☯ Rub the four small toes to help heal the eyesight and hearing.
☯ Rub the feet for mental and physical grounding and physical strength.
☯ Rub your legs to release past problems and to place your mind in the here and now moment.
☯ Rub your buttocks for sciatic nerve problems, relaxation, tension or stress.
☯ Rub the sacrum for lower back pain, hemorrhoids, and menstrual cramps.
☯ Rub your bell (hara) for abundant health and centering, and to gain wisdom, intuition and insight.
☯ Rub in the exact order as outlined above for grounding and centering.

Dao-Yin (Self-Massage) Helps Clear Energy Blockages for Eye and Brain Healing

The basic purpose of Dao-Yin Self-Healing Massage is to break up blockages in the organs, meridians, nerves, muscles, tendons, which increases blood and chi or energy circulation throughout the entire body, including the eyes. When these conditions are met, the body and eyesight automatically receive healing energy. Some of the most vital areas to massage are the neck and solar plexus (hara-belly). The neck, according to Chi Kung Masters, is not only the gateway between the mental and the physical centers, but is also a gateway for the emotional and spiritual centers in the body. A verse in the Bible says: "This wicked and stiff-necked generation..."and the terrible things that were going to happen to them. Mikhael Aivanhov, a Bulgarian Yogi Master states, "The brain and the solar plexus work together. If there is a blockage in the neck and the communication is not very good, you must massage the neck in the region of the cervical vertebrae so as to reestablish the current going from the solar plexus to the brain." This is also important to allow nerve and blood circulation to flow to the tiny nerves and capillaries in the eyes and eye muscles. The eyes actually "see" out through the brain. We actually see with our brain, through the eyes. Vision is really a miraculous phenomenon of Great Nature and the Creative Force of the Universe! Don't you 'see.'

Healing Hara-Belly Massage

The Chinese Dao-Yin healing system recommends that you massage the entire hara (stomach, liver, intestines) from under the rib cage to the pubic bone. Massage deep and slow, with your fingers, knuckles and fist. Massage the entire abdominal area just before bed time, and again before getting out of bed in the morning. When the hara is relaxed during sleep, the internal organs and eyesight are allowed to heal naturally. Plus, we can receive the proper spiritual guidance or intuition for the next day's activity.

The brain and the mind can never have true or correct answers for us, as they are merely intellectual surface tools for everyday life. Zen, Yoga and Taoist Masters' tell their students to "cut off your head"—figuratively, of course! Why? Too much head or brain thinking most always gets us in trouble. We are taught to stop worrying or constantly thinking about our problems. Instead, concentrate and breathe into the lower belly or hara, the center of our being, or God/Tao Center, for peace, guidance, health and happiness.

The Three Power Centers

There are three power centers in the abdomen: 1. The Solar Plexus, in the pit of the abdomen (arch of the rib cage); 2. Behind the belly button area; and, 3. The Dan Tian, 1 1/2 inches below the belly button.

Massage the entire abdomen for a few minutes daily, and you will experience peace, tranquility, self control and answers to your problems. It is also a good idea to receive a 30 to 60 minute hara massage from a massage therapist. In Japan, a Hara Massage

Therapist works on the entire abdomen for an hour or more. Many people experience healing after these intense hara massage sessions. We learned these deep Hara Massage techniques from Chinese and Japanese Dao-Yin and Chi Kung Masters.

The Heart and the Belly

When the ancients talked about the heart, they are talking about the belly or hara. "When initiates speak of the intelligence of the heart," according to Master Aivanhov, "no one, not even the theologians have understood why it is the heart which possesses the veritable intelligence, nor what this intelligence is. To the initiates, the heart is not the pump which propels the blood through the organism, but it is another heart, the Solar Plexus (hara-belly area)."

Dao-Yin is practiced to prevent disease, maintain high-level health, and to cultivate our individual chi energy. Dao-Yin practitioners also use hara massage to help cure illnesses. Ayurvedic and Chinese Medicine both concur that disease begins in the harabelly area (stomach, intestines, liver). Ayurvedic Medicine says: "There is no disease without first gastro-intestinal derangement." Chinese Medicine refers to the Hara-Belly as "Central Energy," where health and energy is generated and maintained. This is also the prime area where disease manifest. For example, when the colon, stomach and liver are functioning below par—weak digestion, fatigue, constipation, diarrhea, hepatitis, diabetes, low blood sugar etc, the eyesight also weakens and becomes diseased.

Oriental Medicine teaches that we must open the blockages in the physical body to receive energy and healing. During an energy imbalance and illness that Robert Zuraw developed several years ago (from Agent Orange Poisoning in Viet Nam, and from eating too much dairy products), he began performing hara-belly massage rubbing. At the time, he overcame his "mysterious illness," and his vision improved every year. There is no limit to how well one can see. With the proper knowledge, understanding and practice, you too can keep your vision for as long as you live. This is really good news. But, you have to take action to follow through on these valuable vision and health training secrets.

Hara Massage for Unlimited Energy

Hara massage is for everyone. Start today on your road to energy and vitality. It is easy and fun to do. It takes about 10 minutes to perform before going to sleep or you can do it in the morning before getting out of bed. It doesn't take much energy to do; in fact, after a few minutes of "belly rubbing" you will feel more energy, along with less stress and nerve exhaustion. Your vision will also improve quicker by performing Hara Massage daily.

Perfect Eyesight

Do not massage the head, ears or eye areas at night, because the energy may go to the head and keep you awake. Perform Dao-Yin head massage in the morning. Always finish a Dao-Yin massage session with a belly massage. This brings the energy to the center of the body, where it creates balance, centeredness and calmness.

Jean Rofidal, writing in "DO.IN: The Philosophy" says, "Many people think they can get by without paying any respect to the rules of the Universal Order, which may be classified under four main headings: nourishment, respiration, exercise and meditation…"they give us the opportunity of doing something about our well being. For instance, by acting on the exterior of our bodies, we can act on the interior and by acting on the gross, we act on the subtle." "Do-In or (Dao-Yin) affords a splendid method of acting on our bodies physically, mentally and spiritually."

Foot Slapping to Invigorate the Kidneys and Nourish the Eyes and Liver
Traditional Chinese Medical Chi Kung Dao-Yin Technique to Improve Mental Health, Energy and Vision

Chi Kung Master Huang Runtian, writing in "Treasured Qigong of Traditional Medical School," states that this "Foot Tapping Technique"…"can nourish the liver and improve eyesight; curing chronic diseases of the liver, gall bladder and eyesight diseases (near-sightedness, far-sightedness, and poor- sightedness)."

"As a result of conscientious practicing of the Qigong exercise, the liver-wood nourished by sufficient kidney-water and abundant "earth Qi" would be full of vigor and vitality. Thus, the Qigong can nourish the liver and make the eyes clear."

"Frequency and duration of this exercise." Slap or clap your feet 50 to 100 times with your cupped hand slowly and deliberately. For health protection, perform once a day before going to bed."

Positive Benefits of Foot Slapping or Tapping

Here are some ailments Chinese Medicine attributes to being helped by foot tapping or slapping: "Yin (cold) deficiency, yang (hot) excess, upper body heat excess, lower body deficiency (ungrounded-ness), kidney and heart problems, excessive rise of liver yang, seminar emissions, night sweats, heart palpitations, poor memory, insomnia, mental

stress, neurasthenia, migraine headaches, knee and back pain, blood deficiency, burning red face, mental depression, poor eyesight, liver and gall bladder problems.

"In practicing Dao-Yin, you need not believe in it, but you must do the exercise earnestly. You will get benefits from it, whether you believe it nor not," says Master Runtian.

Perfect Eyesight

A Personal Experience of Foot Slapping

While visiting Zen-Taoist Master Hyunoong Sunim, in Washington State, I was awakened early one morning by a loud clapping sound. I found out later that he was slapping the bottom of his feet. A few years later, I tested his eyesight, and found that he had better than 20-20 vision. His vision was in the range of 40-10, about three times better than 20-20 normal vision! This was amazing. He could read the 10 foot Snellen Eye Chart at 40 feet away without glasses or contacts! A super feat for someone in his early 40s. The Master also avoided sugar and sweets.

Start practicing Foot Slapping, and make it a daily habit, and watch and feel your energy zoom! This exercise is one of the best Dao-Yin techniques for improving one's health and vision. Begin by slapping each foot only 50 times a day, and work up to 100 and 200, over time. The goal of Foot Slapping is to open up the energy points on the foot, {kidney acupuncture point}, and the energy acupuncture meridian point on the palm, as the palm meets the foot. Once they are opened, over several weeks of practice, foot slapping 50 times before bed will be sufficient. Just relax your palm, and slap at an even slow tempo, about one second for each slap.

Overcoming Depression and Emotional Problems with Foot Slapping

Traditional Chinese Medicine (TCM) talks about those who suffer from an *excess* of the seven human emotions—joy, anger, anxiety, worry, grief, apprehension and fear. These emotions, in excess, are the cause of much depression and emotional diseases. We have an epidemic of mental illnesses, depression and emotional problems in the world today. These illnesses can be a direct cause of poor health and faulty vision.

Taoist's call these mental problems "sentimental diseases." Sentimental diseases are caused by the misuse or abuse of the emotions. These emotional illnesses are based on negative emotions. For example, people die of an excess of grief. Hair can turn white overnight from an excess of fear or stress. Losing a job or a break-up of a relationship has caused many to stay depressed for years—also causing headaches, bulimia, anorexia and crying spells. Worry causes spleen and stomach illness, and poor digestion. Diarrhea or a weak bladder can be caused by fright. Heart attacks have happened after "winning" at the race track. Anxiety and fear has kept many from success, with its paralyzing effect. Excess anger can cause strokes, liver problems and weak vision. These are examples of "sentimental diseases."

The Hara, Brain Activity and Visual Clarity

We use our brain machine far too much to our own detriment, unlike our ancient ancestors, who had slower brain activity, no technology; less worry and anxiety, and less intellectual thinking. Excessive thinking and negative emotions moves our energy up to the head, instead of down in the Hara-Belly area, where it needs to be to stay calm. The Hara and Solar Plexus is called the second brain, where we get our "gut" feelings or intuition. When our mind is confused, visual clarity also drop dramatically.

Most of us refuse to see that we caused our own problems in the first place, by making emotional or irrational decisions.

Balancing Upper and Lower Body Centers

Because we overuse our brains, we are more strongly afflicted with the "seven negative sentimental emotions." As a result we suffer from an excess of energy in the upper body, and a deficiency in the lower body, especially the Hara-Belly area. Be reversing this energy pattern, we can restore our balance between the Yin lower), and the Yang (upper) part of the body to increase our health and vision.

We can overcome these imbalanced negative mental states, and balance our head with our hara, by making healthy food choices and performing Hara Massage and Foot Slapping daily.

How to Perform the Foot Slapping Dao-Yin Technique to Strengthen the Kidneys and Adjust Your Energy Levels

The regular practice of this Foot Slapping Dao-Yin Technique has proven in Traditional Chinese Medicine to renew physical and mental health and help to restore good health, vision and long life, along with a healthy lifestyle program.

Foot Slapping Technique

Step One: Sit on a chair, close eyes, relax body
Step Two: Breathe naturally. Rid the mind of distractions. Be silent for a few minutes.
Step Three: Open eyes. Place right foot on left knee.
Step Four: With open palm, slap the arch of the right foot with the palm of the left hand. In the palm is located the "laogong Point" acupoint. This acupoint on the foot is called the Yongquan Point. **(See Figure 1-5).** The middle of the hand acupoint, (Laogong) is slapped on the top arch of the foot—Yongquan Acupoint.

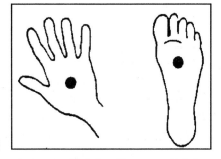

Figure 1-5

Laogong Point   Yongqua Point

Step Five: While slapping the foot, hit with an even force and a relaxed tempo—with cupped **palm—not too hard, but medium. Do not slap your foot with a stiff or rigid hand. Keep your** wrist area loose and relaxed while slapping. Do the same with the other foot.
Step Six: Meditate or be silent for a few minutes.

Step Seven: Frequency: Slap your foot at least 50 times morning and night. Work up to 100 times.

Perfect Eyesight

Point of Attention

If you are a beginner at foot slapping, go easy—do not cause yourself pain or soreness. Just slap your foot gently for the first 2 weeks. Take it easy and relax into it. Increase the force as you improve. Once the Acupoint is opened, the sting, soreness or redness will no longer be there. After the Point is opened, do only 50 slaps before bed.

If you have low-blood pressure or hypoglycemia, place one hand on the top of your head, while the other hand slaps your foot. Do not practice foot slapping if you suffer from a serious health problem or are extremely weak, i.e., cancer or heart conditions. For the seriously ill, just rub the foot and finish by rubbing the belly a few minutes.

Foot Slapping Balances Water and Fire in the Body

For good health, the body requires that water moves upward and fire moves downward. This is because the head and brain must remain cool and calm, while the hands and feet remain warm. When one is ill, the head is usually hot with fire, and the hands and feet are cool, cold or clammy and moist.

Slapping the bottom of the feet brings the fire down and helps the water go up. Good health requires that we maintain sufficient Kidney-Chi Energy, which means strong well-functioning kidneys. When the Kidney Yongquan Point is opened you will be able to draw the energy of the earth into your body (earth magnetism). Slapping the Yongquan Point can also help those who have performed chi kung incorrectly or who have had an energy blockage (chi energy not flowing smoothly throughout the body)—constant nausea, headaches, dizziness, hot head, cold hands, ear ringing etc.

Foot slapping harmonizes the heart and kidneys. When the kidneys become healthy and vigorous, they nourish the liver, which also improves and enhances the eyesight for near and far vision. Start practicing this Foot Slapping Technique today and feel your health and energy zoom! Let us hear of your progress as you continue to practice these special oriental Chi Kung and Dao Yin Self-Healing Techniques, and other vision exercises in this book. Now turn to **Chapter Six**, and get ready to discover the real inner Nutritional Secrets to improve your vision beyond the ordinary!

Chapter Six
Nutritional Secrets for Visual Clarity

Healing Your Eyesight and Body with Whole Foods

Good nutrition is vitally important in your quest for strong and healthy eye muscles, nerves and blood vessels. These eye components determine the health and vitality of our vision. If you are weak, tired or run-down, with dull unclear vision, malnutrition or mal-absorption of vital food nutrients is the immediate cause.

Health and nutrition is your own personal responsibility. How you eat determines your state of health. If you eat devitalized foods, you develop a 'devitalized' body, and your eyes become dim and lifeless. Hypocrites, the father of modern medicine, once stated that: "Your food shall be your medicine, and your medicine shall be your food."

Food is our direct link to Mother Earth. Natural food gives us natural chemical elements called minerals, vitamins, enzymes, fiber, trace elements and organic liquid. These are the life-giving elements that feed cells, tissues, hair, skin, bones, teeth and eyes. Without a daily flow of these powerful little dynamos in your system, you can forget about good health and Perfect Eyesight!

Make nutrition, health and fitness your daily routine and habit. Health should be your first and foremost hobby. Is a car, house, boat, or expensive "toys" more important than the health of your most important possession—you and your loved ones!?

"Physician, Heal Thyself."

Who is this "Physician?" **You Are!** If you seek good health and perfect eyesight, only YOU can give yourself the necessary understanding to apply the laws of nutrition to your Divine Temple!

Only you can know how to flow with the natural rhythm of life—when you are hungry, tired, sleepy, thirsty etc. Only you can know when to eat when you have 'true hunger,' rest when tired, sleep when sleepy, drink when thirsty, exercise when full of energy, meditate when the spirit moves you and eliminate when 'nature calls,' etc. When you pay attention to your 'original nature'--internal physiological needs, intuitive feelings—you will be led to a 'natural' moderation in all your activities.

Learn to eat correctly, and your health, vision and energy will zoom with rocket-like power. Eyes are the most abused organ in the body. They reflect the condition of the body organs—good or poor, especially, the liver and gall bladder. These two organs work together to detox the body of excess chemicals, fats, junk food and environmental poisons.

If one has a weak, malfunctioning liver and gall bladder, the eyes may show some of these symptoms and characteristics: aching eyes, headache in the forehead area, bloodshot eyes, yellow eye whites, jaundiced eyes, excess bulging eyes, watery eyes, eye spots, itching eyes etc.

Discover the Inner Secrets of Health, Nutrition and Unlimited Energy Through.......

The Five Health-Nutrition Keys to Perfect Eyesight

Health Key Number One
Eat only when hungry and drink liquids only when thirsty.

It is said that 'Very few people die from starvation, but millions die prematurely from over-eating.' Another wise jokester stated: "Half the food we eat feeds us, the other half feeds the doctor."

The stomach, which houses the digestive system, operates like a pot belly stove. Over-stuff a pot-belly stove with wood, and you get nothing but smoke; it refused to burn smoothly. But, fill the same stove 3/4 full and the wood burns beautifully. Your stomach will also not burn (digest) food smoothly if you stuff it to the "gills," with food. Eat food to one-half or 3/4 full & stop! Health and energy follows those that heed this advice.

Perfect Eyesight

Eating too soon after a previous meal is also a poor health habit. Stuffing one meal too soon before the last one has completely digested, always results in putrefaction and fermentation, which causes indigestion and toxemia—a loss of nerve energy, fatigue and further ill-health. Overeating destroys the nutritional value of the food eaten.

Even whole, natural food will not digest properly if you stuff your 'stove.' Eating when not hungry and over-eating leads to malnutrition and poor eyesight.

There is an inner physiological voice within you, that tells you when, what and how much you need to eat everyday. Listen to your body intelligence. What do you feel? Are you really hungry? Or do you eat out of boredom, depression or emotions?

What are the physical and psychological signs of hunger? Your mouth should water. Tongue is pink, watery and clear—no white, yellow, green, brown or black coating. Tongue coating indicates that undigested food has not evacuated the stomach, small intestines or colon. The tongue is the upper gateway to the lower gastrointestinal system. Hunger is a mouth and throat sensation—not stomach pangs. Stomach grumbling or pangs indicates toxins or undigested food in the stomach, It is also an indication that one has over-indulged in excessively stimulating foods and drinks, meat, dairy products, processed foods, sugar, candy, cake, pop, alcohol, and other commercial junk food.

Positive sign of true hunger: If you are truly hungry, you will be happy, joyous, with a real yearning for food when true hunger is present at mealtimes. Your energy should also be high before eating. Tiredness, fatigue, emotional upsets and stress is not a good time to eat. Rest 30-60 minutes first, then eat when your energy is restored. Food digests smoothly and completely when one is rested and full of energy and vitality. In fact, indigestion is one of the greatest causes of energy loss, disease and poor eyesight. *The immune system is directly connected to the power and efficiency of good digestion, assimilation, absorption and elimination of food. The Gut area (hara) is called Central Energy in Chinese Medicine, and is the key to restoring health in a sick body!*

There is a saying "Eat to live–not live to eat." Most people live only to see how much they can stuff down their gullet. They live only for "mouth amusement," or to tickle their "taste-buds." Food must be delicious, nutritious and tasteful, but don't obsess over it. If you eat wholesome, nutritious foods, you will be satisfied on less food—and be better nourished. If food is digested and assimilated well—with no stomach aches, indigestion or gas—the eyes receive a good flow of micro-nutrients and you will experience better results while performing your eye exercises.

Important Health Note: **Eat only when hungry. 'When you know when enough is enough, you will always have enough." –Taoism**

Perfect Eyesight

Health Key Number Two
Chew Your Food Well. Your Key to Good Eyesight and Health

Observe the 12 noon lunch hour at the office. The robot-like machines rush from their desks to the nearest "fast-food greasy-spoon slop-house." The food is gulped and swallowed like swine-in-swill. No thought is taken as to what kind of so-called food or drink goes into their sacred Body-Temple. All of this lifeless junk food is then washed down with a large sugared drink, coffee or tea. How can you build good health, energy and good eyesight with these non-nutritious foods and poor eating habits? Fast foods lead to fast diseases and a fast trip to the cemetery. Like anything else in life, disease is a "process" that one builds over time. It is the effect of ill habits of eating and living, and the end process is disease and suffering.

Humans eat fast. There is so much work to do. "I rush back to my office, and by 3 or 4 pm, I am exhausted and stressed out. I reach for another coffee and donut to boost my sagging spirit." Ayurvedic Wisdom says: "There is no disease, without first, gastro-intestinal derangement."

This scenario goes on every day in every big city in the world. And the hospitals and morgues are filled with such sad souls who didn't take the time to chew, relax, digest, assimilate, meditate and contemplate on where the food came from, where they are going on this mud-ball, and what life is all about.

Food gulped down on the run cannot possibly be digested properly. Proper chewing sets our digestive juices flowing. It gets the food ready for thorough assimilation in the gastro-intestinal tract and healthy bowel elimination. Bowel problems start with poor eating habits.

Eating too fast prevents good digestion; consequently, the food lays in the stomach and immediately putrefies and ferments. So, you hear 'gas-wars' going on in millions of offices throughout the land. We have no real gas shortage! Scientists should find a way to hook-up 'that gas' to run our cities' electrical power!

It all gets back to chewing. Chewing is an art. Why? Because our stomach has no teeth to handle un-chewed food. Although, I did hear of a man who swallowed his false teeth. So, he could gulp his food and chew later! Seriously, digestion starts with the saliva in the mouth with the enzyme ptyalin. Ptyalin breaks down starch in the mouth before entering the stomach for further digestion. We by-pass the first step of digestion when we gulp and run. Long-lived people always chew their food slowly–20-30 times per mouthful. Macrobiotics say: "Chew fine, think fine. Chew rough, think rough." Enjoy the taste of your food; this makes your digestive juices flow smoothly, and enables you to utilize the essential nutritional ingredients of the food for improved eyesight and good health.

Health Key Number Three
Eat Mostly Whole Natural Foods in Season and In Your Climate

The optimum diet for Perfect Eyesight, health and longevity is one that includes plenty of whole grains (rice, barley, millet, rye, wheat, oats, buckwheat, spelt, amaranth, kamut and pasta made from them), vegetables (lightly steamed in winter and raw in summer).

Supplement this basic Whole Foods Diet with some raw fruits eaten mostly in warm summer months. Nuts and seeds should be soaked in water overnight to revive their life-force, or use them in soups and cooking: almonds, walnuts, cashews, sesame seeds, sunflower and pumpkin seeds; beans (green and yellow split peas, aduki, navy, kidney, black, garbanzo, lentils, lima etc.; If you are not a vegetarian, keep your animal foods (organic source), to no more than 5-!0% of your diet, to maintain a proper alkaline/acid balance and good health. Vegans can eat seeds, beans, hemp seeds, rice protein powder, quinoa and tempeh for protein.

Alaskan, Australian or New Zealand fish is virtually mercury and chemical free. All other fish from large coastal cities are highly contaminated. Organic chicken and turkey are better than commercial brands. Organic eggs and milk far surpass commercial variety in quality and nutrients. Five to 10% animal products will give you sufficient protein to maintain your body in good health.

If you want to feel and look your best, consume foods that are grown within a 500 mile radius of where you live, and eat them in their proper season. That means eat seasonal fruits and vegetables when they are harvested in your area. In Michigan, asparagus comes out in May. Early leafy greens come out in June. Berries in June and July. Melons and corn in August and September. Apples in September and October etc.

Tender fresh raw fruits and vegetables come out in the Spring and Summer for a reason. They cleanse the liver of toxins that accumulated during the winter months. Berries, especially blueberries, blackberries, strawberries, raspberries, cherries help to detox the liver, cleanse the blood and increase iron and oxygen in the system. Asparagus, dandelion greens, lettuce, and spinach are also good choices to get green chlorophyll into your body.

Soaked and cooked grains, beans, soups, pasta, steamed root vegetables are more suitable for cold winter months to impart strength and maintain heat in the body, hands, feet. Remember: Raw food is loaded with potassium–a cooling mineral to cool the blood and body during hot summer months. Cooked whole foods, on the other hand, are higher in sodium, phosphorus, nitrogen–warming minerals to warm-up the blood and body in cold winter months.

If you listen to your intuition (body intelligence), it will lead you to the right foods for the right climate and season. Get tested occasionally by a qualified wholistic health doctor to check for proper Vitamin D, Calcium, Iron, B-Vitamins, Hormones and Thyroid levels.

Health Key Number Four
Super-Nutrient-Rich Foods for Perfect Eyesight

Seeds contain the life-giving force of nature bundled-up in a tiny package. Seeds are the beginning of another life. They come from life and they give us life when we eat them. Soak all seeds, nuts, grains and beans overnight in water to get rid of the enzyme inhibitors and phytic acids that these products contain in their dry state. The soaking process takes out the acids, and makes these products more alkaline, thereby helping you to digest them better, for improved health and energy.

Sunflower seeds are a supreme food for the eyes. They contain Vitamin B-2 which helps to prevent an overcome photo-phobia (fear of light). They are also high in Vitamin D, the sunshine vitamin. The sunflower seed plant turns its head to the Sun, thereby absorbing the glorious life-giving Solar Orb. Eat a tablespoon of sunflowers daily in your cereal, soaked overnight and notice how you can easily take sunlight or headlight glare.

Carrots or carrot juice works wonders for night vision. Carrots are high in vitamin A. The body does not require a high intake of Vitamin A daily, because it is stored in the liver for future use. So, a 4-6 ounce glass of carrot juice, or five carrots a week is enough to give you plenty of beta-carotene and vitamin A for sparkling clear vision.

Edgar Cayce, the "Sleeping Prophet", speaks highly of carrots as a remedy for many ailments in his dietary remedy books.

We recommend eating only organic carrots. Unlike the commercial, chemicalized variety, organic carrots are naturally sweet and delicious. They are loaded with over four times the vitamins, minerals, trace elements and healing power as the anemic chemical brand. Carrots are noted for soaking up whatever is in the soil. Guess what? You guessed it! Commercial carrots are packed full of health-destroying chemical fertilizers, pesticides, and the latest brand of devastating immune-system-destroying chemical sprays. However, our gracious Mother Earth will have the last word on this! She may be getting ready to rumble and shake-up the sleeping mechanical robots who are choking Her life-roots with toxic chemical poisons!

Eat organic vegetables and carrots, and be on the safe side. Mother Nature and Mother Earth will place you in Her protective arms if you follow Her Natural Laws of food, eating and health.

Herbs to Heal and Protect Your Liver and Vision

Blueberries, bilberry and raspberry herb teas are all good for night vision. Parsley contains Vitamin B-2, which helps to improve day visio
Eyebright herb tea has been used for centuries for improving the eyesight. Steep a teaspoon of eyebright in hot water for 20 minutes and drink a cup a day. Dandelion *root* tea improves distant vision (nearsightedness). Dandelion *leaf* tea helps you to see better close (farsightedness).

Perfect Eyesight

Chinese Lychii (gogi) berries and Chrysanthemum are highly acclaimed in the orient for promoting better vision and reducing liver toxicity. Use lychii (goji) berry and chrysanthemum for a month, then change to the Western herbs—eyebright and dandelion the following month.

Licorice root is an excellent herb to reduce inflammation, mucous and to improve vision. Use no more than a 1/4 teaspoon of licorice powder with water daily. Or chew on a small piece of licorice stick. Ayurvedic physician, Dr. Vinod Verma, recommends to: "Take [licorice] as a preventative measure after age 35, as many people tend to get problems with their vision around that age." Licorice is said to increase one's memory and mental clarity.

Foods that Heal, Cleanse and Strengthen the Liver and Eyes

Here is a list of vegetables, fruits and seeds to strengthen and heal your liver, eyes and immune system: Yams, squash, potatoes carrots, beets, dandelion greens, celery, cabbage, broccoli, chard, kale, collards, green beans, fresh snow peas & green peas, blueberries, raspberries, mangos, grapefruit, sunflower seeds, pumpkin seeds, all radishes, mushrooms, kombucha tea, Blue Green Algae, Green Kamut, Spirulina, Green Barley Magma. Also, include all the other vegetables in your diet for variety. Green vegetables help to clear the eyes and prevent eye inflammation. Grains contain Vitamin B-Complex, which strengthens eye nerves and the entire nervous system. It imparts steady nerves and steady eyes. Buckwheat contains *rutin* to repair and heal cells and tissues. Barley and barley greens helps to heal tumors and inflammations. Oatmeal is rich in *silicon* for sparkling eyes, lustrous hair and strong nails.

Health Key Number Five
Toxic Foods that Cause Ill Health and Vision Problems

Did you know that the average "American diet" is costing us over 900 billion dollars yearly in medical bills! We are consuming 150 pounds of refined white sugar, 85 pounds of processed oils and fats, 150 pounds of white flour, 15 pounds of white rice, cases of alcohol and thousands of cigarettes per person annually! In the early 1900s, Americans ate only 5 pounds of white sugar per person. Today that statistic is 125 pounds per person yearly.

Disease is on the rise. Hospitals are filled to capacity. Jails and mental institutions are over-crowded. Three-fourths of the population suffers from poor health, poor vision, require eye glasses and eventually eye surgery! This is a tragic statistic. As a nation, we are going down-hill fast. This shows the power of mass hypnotism, via the media—TV, papers, radio—concerning our health or lack thereof. Junk foods, medicines, alcohol and fast living are all promoted by large corporations, with little regard for our health, sanity or well-being. Many people are walking around today in a "somnambulistic trance," (as G. Gurdjieff once said), addicted to material things, power, greed, fast foods, sugared drinks, drugs, coffee, cigarettes and alcohol! Where it will end, no one knows. Only **YOU** can take charge of your life, health and eyesight. If you practice these teachings, you will enjoy your life in peace, health and happiness. We can only set an example for others, who are ready to follow.

Perfect Eyesight

Medical doctors are now finding a close link between dietary habits and disease causation. Holistic doctors have known about this for centuries. In the early 1900s only six-percent of the population was nearsighted. Today, over 65 percent have eye problems!

Good health and good eyesight go hand in hand. Avoid junk foods and poisons: chemical drug medications, antibiotics, white sugar, pops, candy, cakes etc., commercial milk (loaded with bovine growth hormones, steroids etc.), white table salt, white refined flour (bread, pastries etc.), solid fats (lard) cheap supermarket vegetable oils (extremely rancid, canola oil, soy oil, vegetable margarine (made from hydrogenated oils), high salt foods, commercial butter, dairy, yogurt, milk and cheese. These are all loaded with growth hormones and antibiotics. Shop at your local health store for higher quality products. They usually stock organic dairy products. However, read the labels; not everything in a health store is healthy or low-fat, or good fat. **Buyer beware!** Go easy on the dairy, as it contains lactose, which is hard to digest.

Sugar Blues, Depression and Myopia (Nearsightedness)

Sugar is clearly the most deadly food for your eyesight! This also includes raw brown sugar, which is just white sugar with molasses added for coloring. Don't be fooled by this gimmick.

Sugar robs all the bones and teeth of calcium and the all important B-vitamins; it destroys the pancreas—uses up insulin and causes diabetes, obesity, heart disease, skin diseases, poor memory, kidney and liver disorders and poor eyesight. Sugar forms a "crystalline lens" on the eyes, causing cataracts; it is the main cause of inflamed eyes.

Dr. Jin Otsuka, a leading Japanese authority on nearsightedness says "If you feed sugar to a rabbit, the rabbit becomes myopic (nearsighted). Even so-called natural sugars, like honey, maple syrup, rice syrup, barley malt etc., eaten in excess, weakens the organs and causes poor vision.

The human body only produces one tablespoon of insulin daily. If you drink a large glass of carrot juice or fruit juice, and two tablespoons of honey, you have just used-up your supply of insulin for the day. Consume four or five times more than this every day for years, and you create hypoglycemia (low blood sugar) and finally diabetes (no insulin produced in the pancreas).

Simple mathematics! Weaken the organs with excess sugars, fats, refined flour, drugs, alcohol etc., and you're left with zero health. Nothing left in the balance. Hormones dry up and disappear. No hormones, no health. No health, no life—period! Got it!

If you seek high energy every day, then you'll have to limit your intake of natural sweets, like honey, maple syrup to two or three teaspoons daily—no more. Limit your intake of juices also. Fruit juices are concentrated sugars, extracted from the whole fruit. If you need juice, dilute it 3/4 with water. You'll save your organs from overworking.

Excess sweets further weakens the adrenal glands, which give us energy during the day. Eat some fruit, especially in warm summer weather. Fruits are good organ cleansers and contain oxygen and iron for blood building. Fruit is high in potassium (a cooling mineral), so reduce its consumption in cold winter weather. The body doesn't need a lot of potassium in the winter. You can, however, occasionally stew or cook some fruit in cool weather if you are healthy. More fruit in hot summer, less in winter.

Excess Salt and Weak Vision

Excessive salt consumption leads to hardening of the arteries, high blood pressure, obesity etc. Hardened arteries causes poor circulation to the eyes and weak vision. Excess salt congests the kidneys and eventually creates edema (waterlogged body). Use kelp or powdered vegetable seasoning instead of common table salt. Instead, use Celtic Salt or Himalayan Salt—they contain many more trace minerals. A pinch will do.

White Flour and Poor Vision

White flour when mixed with the digestive juices becomes a paste, like 'Plaster of Paris.' We become glued-up inside. Literally, blocked-up or constipated from these "refined foods." Many people walk around with 15 to 20 pounds of dried-up fecal matter pasted up against their colon walls. Not a happy camper! You see these type of angry people driving down the road giving out "middle-finger hand signals" to other 'slow' motorists!

Ayurvedic medicine from India teaches that constipation must be overcome in order to improve the eyesight. Constipation is a direct cause of blurred, dim vision, and many major diseases. "There is no disease, without first gastro-intestinal derangement."

Fats and Oils in the Blood

You'll feel great if you keep your fat intake around 5% to 10% of your diet Go easy on these high fat foods: Milk, cheese, butter, dairy, oils, meats. Eat them sparingly or go on a Vegan diet, and watch your health improve. Excess consumption of fats cannot be digested, assimilated and absorbed completely, which results in higher blood cholesterol and blocked arteries, liver and gall bladder stones. This slows down the circulation to the eyes, as well as to the heart and other major internal organs. Nuts and nut butters, eaten to excess, can also congest the liver and cause inflammation and poor vision.

Fats are also implicated in diabetes, obesity and liver disease. The liver and gall bladder metabolize fats. Gall stones are caused from an excess of animal fats in the diet. In the Chinese Five Element System, the liver rules the eyes. So, a fatty liver causes many eye disorders, i.e., jaundice, dark spots, yellow eyes, red eyes, blindness, astigmatism, crossed eyes and poor vision etc. Junk foods are causing many

Perfect Eyesight

degenerative diseases throughout the world. You can avoid eye problems by eating plenty of whole foods, herbs and performing your eye routine a couple times a week.

Dangerous Oils that Destroy Vision

Some vegetable oils are better than others for health and longevity. First, the bad news oils.

HEALTH WARNING NOTE! **If you desire good vision and super-health avoid, like the plague, all these oils, foods with these oils in them and their by-products: All vegetable margarine: cotton seed oil, oleo-margarine, margarine made from corn oil, safflower, soy oil and canola oil. Soy and Canola are industrial oils and extremely toxic in the human body! Use these oils to grease your car only!**

All margarine is hydrogenated and **solid** at room temperature, which makes it saturated. Oils are boiled at extremely high temperatures through a nickel alloy, which makes it hard at room temperature on your dinner table! Margarine will harden your arteries in a jiffy, and cut your life in half. We call it "plastic fat." Avoid it and live healthy and long!

GMO Non-Organic Soybean Products CAN Cause Toxic Blood and Weak Vision

Soy is a poisonous weed grown for human and animal consumption. Bugs will not eat soy plants, because they detect poison in the plant. People and animals get sick on the stuff. Animals that eat a lot of soy products live only half their normal age. When I ate soy hot dogs, tofu, soy margarine, soy powders, my eyes and health were below par. You can feel the difference in energy by cutting out soy. Organic tempeh, miso and other fermented organic soy products are fine to eat occasionally. Fermented soy is easy to digest, and does not contain enzyme inhibitors and phytates.

Soy and canola are considered negative or left-spin energy plants. They can grow on "diseased" soil and air. They take in and store the toxic environment (chemical-laden dead soils and polluted air) inside the beans. Hard salt fertilizers and poisonous sprays are used to produce the toxic soy bean. Unbelievable, but true! Other healthy natural foods such as grains, beans, vegetables, fruit, seeds, nuts, are called "positive" or right-spin energy plant foods. Positive energy plant foods do not disrupt or damage health and vitality. Eighty to 90% of all soy products are Genetically Modified(GMO).

Fermented cultured soy, like tempeh, miso or tamari soy sauce and fermented soy powder are not harmful, but make sure they are non-GMO and organically produced.

In the mid-50s soy beans were "irradiated" to increase their oil content. This in-turn produced more oil on "negative energy soils." "Soy oil is an 'industrial' oil, not a food oil!" This is a serious matter, if you desire good health and clear vision. Don't take it lightly.

Oils, Vision Defects, Balding and Immune System Deficiencies

Balding, eye problems, liver problems, yeast infections, poor digestion, fatigue etc., are closely linked with the use of these dangerous oils. Tofu, soy 'hot dogs', soy milk, and soy burgers fall into the same disease-causing category. These products all cause premature old age! How is that, you say?

Cows that graze on soy die quickly. Hair quickly "falls out" on sheep that graze on soy plants. Dr. Carry Reams found "a link between the soybean, balding, and deterioration in the blood." Soy oil, soy products and tofu contain a poisonous chemical called "phyto-hema-glutinin" or PHG. It is a large protein molecule that causes the blood to clot or stick together like glue, forming plaques on the arterioles, that clog the capillaries in the eyes, ears and scalp, causing eye problems, ear infections and hair loss.

Soy oil and canola oil products weaken the immune system's T cells, weakening the nervous and hormonal systems. PHG in soy and canola kills small rodents fast. These products are systemic toxins, accumulating slowly, causing many disease conditions.

Vegetarians Beware of GMO and Isolated Soy Products

Vegetarians must especially be wary of eating "isolated" soy food products, like unfermented soy isolate "protein" powders, soy milk, soy cheese, soy tofu, as all of these foods contain high amounts of phytic acids, that can bind up minerals in the body. Phytates are also enzyme inhibitors, which hinder proper digestion of proteins, complex carbohydrates in the GI tract, causing indigestion, bloating, poor absorption and poor health. Instead, use cultured and fermented soy products, like tempeh, miso, fermented soy powders, organic soy sauce, plain soy yogurt, which are easily digested, assimilated, and their phytate and enzyme inhibitor problem is removed. Also, avoid fake "cheese" substitutes made from almonds, soy, rice—all high in canola, soy oil, and highly processed. Tofu is loaded with mostly water and is a poor protein source, difficult to digest, assimilate, absorb and eliminate. Soybeans undergo hours of processing, cooking and preparing to make "cheese" and tofu. They weaken the immune system, thyroid function and absorption of many vitamins, minerals and enzymes in the body. Eat a variety of fermented foods listed above, plus sauerkraut, pickles, sourdough bread, pickled beets etc. Plenty of friendly bacteria here.

(See Appendix I: 20 Keys to Health and Longevity).

The Ill-Effects of Rapeseed-Canola Oil and Soy Oil on Liver, Blood, Eyes and Health
by John Thomas, Author of *"Young Again!"*

The name Canola is a "coined" word. Canola oil comes from the rape seed, which is part of the Mustard family of plants. Rape seed is the **MOST** toxic of all food oil plants. It is not listed in anything but the most recent reference sources. It is a word that appeared out of *nowhere*. Canola oil is a semi-drying oil that is used as a lubricant, fuel, soap, rubber products and magazine covers. Canola forms latex-like substances that cause **agglutination** of the red blood corpuscles, as does soy only MUCH more pronounced.

Loss of vision is a **known characteristic** side effect of of rape oil. Rape (Canola) antagonizes the central and peripheral nervous systems--like soy oil, only worse. **Rape (Canola) oil causes pulmonary emphysema, respiratory distress, anemia, constipation, irritability and blindness in the bodies of animals, and humans.**

Rape seed oil was in widespread use in animal feeds in England and Europe between 1986 and 1991 when it was thrown out. Do you remember reading about the cows, pigs, and sheep that went **blind,** lost their minds, and attacked people? They had to be shot! ...the "experts" blamed the erratic behavior on a viral disease called "scrapie." However, when rape oil was removed from animal feed, "Scrapie" disappeared. **Now we are growing rape seed and using rape (canola) oil in the USA!** Canola oil is now *our* problem. It is widely used in thousands of processed foods in the USA—with the blessings of government watch-dog agencies, of course!

Officially, canola oil is known as "LEAR" oil. The acronym stands for *low erucic acid* **rape.** The experts tell us it is "safe" to use. Through *genetic engineering i.e.,* irradiation, it is no longer rape, but instead "canola!" The experts talk about canola's "qualities"—like its unsaturated structure, omega 3, 6 and 12, its wonderful digestibility, and its fatty acid makeup. They turn us against naturally saturated oils and fats...The term *canola* provided the perfect cover for commercial interests who wanted to make billions in the USA. The name "canola" is still in use, but it is no longer needed...look at the peanut butter ingredient labels. The peanut oil has been removed and replaced with **rape** oil. Rape oil is used to produce the chemical warfare agent, "MUSTARD GAS," used in all wars, including the recent Gulf War.

Canola oil contains large amounts of **"iso-thio-cyanates'** which are **cyanide** compounds. Cyanide INHIBITS mitochondrial production of ATP. ATP powers the body and keeps us healthy and YOUNG! Notice the tremendous increase in disorders like systemic lupus, multiple sclerosis, cerebral palsy, myelinoma, pulmonary hypertension, and neuropathy in recent years. Soy and canola oils are players in the development of these disease conditions. Canola oil is rich in glycosides which cause serious problems in the human body by blocking enzyme function and depriving us of our life force, Chi, Prana.

Soy and canola oil glycosides depress the immune system. They cause the **white blood cell defense system—the the T-cells**—to go into a stupor and fall asleep on the job. These oils alter the bio-electric "terrain" and promote disease. The alcohols and glycosides in canola and soy oils shut down our protective grid—the immune system.

In the Movie "Lorenzo's Oil"...the dying boy had a chronically low total body pH! So low that his body fluids were *dissolving* the myelin sheath that protects the nerve fibers. causing his nervous system to *disintegrate.* The boy was given Lorenzo's oil to boost energy output and act as a detoxifier of metabolic poisons. The oil shocked his body into a LESS acid condition. Lorenzo's oil is OLIVE OIL! When given in large quantities, olive oil SHOCKS the body and causes it to adjust its pH. It will also SAFELY purge the body of gall and liver stones, thus avoiding the need for gallbladder surgery (Yucca extract and PAC's must precede the "flush." ...On a TV talk show, an "expert" claimed that Lorenzo's oil was rape oil. THIS WAS A LIE! Give rape oil to a sick person and you will seal their doom. Here is another example of "disinformation" in the public domain. These falsehoods should cause every thinking person to question the molding of public opinion by powerful commercial interests behind the scenes....the astronomical increase in the use of processed foods that contain canola oil, soy oil, and chemical additives CONFUSES the body and weakens the immune system. Consuming whole organic natural foods and using Systemic Herbal Formulas can bring your body system back to balance. (See www.systemicformulas.com).

The "health care" industry is an OXYMORON. It protects its own economic interests. If you want peak health and longevity you MUST take control of your life, and be responsible for your health. There is NO other way! Order "Young Again" ($1995) from Promotion Publishing 3368 F Governor Dr. Ste 144,San Diego, CA 92121, or call: 800-231-1776.

Non-Organic, Non-Fermented Soy Isolates Cause of Deranged Digestion

Soybeans can cause weak digestion, gas and a deranged body chemistry in many vegetarians and sensitive people. Peanuts contain only a small amount of PHG in comparison to soybeans and some people cannot digest peanut butter. Use of these products can speed-up mental deterioration in young or old people, ultimately causing Alzheimer's. "Phyto-hema-glutinin" or PHG is contained in the oil of soybeans or tofu. If you use fat-free or oil-free soy products, the health-destroying effects are greatly reduced.

What about soy protein powder or tofu? Tofu is difficult to digest for most people. Eaten excessively, soy products weaken the gastro-intestinal and immune systems. Liver and kidney function are also greatly impaired. If you are sick, weak, fatigued or cancerous, avoid soy and tofu completely. If you have poor digestion, gas or bloating, forget about soy products altogether.

Genetically Modified Soy Protein is Not a Growth Protein

The Net Protein Utilization (NPU) of soy products is a low 10-15 percent. Far too low to maintain good digestion and overall health. The raw soy protein is almost indigestible. Animals fed raw soy plants become ill and die. Dogs, cats and other household pets fed a steady diet of soy tofu and soy products develop illnesses and live to only four to six years old. Non-GMO fermented and cultured organic soy products will not cause these problems. (It is best to get tested with bio-feedback or acupuncture meridian reading machines to determine if you are sensitive to soy foods, or any other foods. "The Compass" by Zyto measures 75 acupuncture meridian body points to determine organ, and health problems, and makes recommendation for herbs, foods, and supplements to balance health). If your digestion is weak avoid unfermented soy.

"Free" amino acid soy proteins are a positive right spin energy product and is acceptable to eat, because their "negative" vibration is neutralized—their oil is removed completely. These are cultured plain soy yogurt, organic tempeh, miso and tamari.

<u>Important Health Note on Oils, Caution!</u>: **Read labels and watch for soy, canola, cotton-seed oil in thousands of food products! These toxic oils do not belong in the human blood system. They get sticky inside the body, cause clotting, blocked arteries and untold damage to our health. Peanut oil is better on the skin then inside the body. Cotton seed oil is known to lower testosterone and sperm count in males! Men beware of cotton seed oil, soy and canola oils in many snacks, chips, health candies, corn chips etc. Read labels. Get informed. Take charge of your own health and healing!**

Also, avoid oils that deteriorate and become rancid quickly, i.e., almond, corn, safflower, avocado, peanut, (peanut oil and peanut butter is also loaded with PHG, and will make your blood clot and become gluey. Instead, **use the healthy oils listed next.**

Use Healthy Oils Moderately for Good Vision and Health
The Best Oils: Olive, Sesame, Sunflower, Flax

Olive is the Rolls Royce of oils! It comes from a fruit--the olive. Other 'right spin positive energy oils are **sesame, sunflower, grapeseed, coconut, and flax.** Vegans can use these healthful vegetable oils. Coconut oil/butter is a medium chain fatty acid and excellent for your health, in spite of the dairy industry's campaign to give it a bad name. These oils are more stable and do not break down as fast as the "bad oils." Keep all oils refrigerated after opening, except coconut oil—it can stay out and not go bad indefinitely! Other oils maintain their freshness in the fridge. Do not consume excessive oils, even the good ones. A tablespoon or two in cooking or on salads is enough to lubricate your glands, hormones and joints. Remember: You are not a car--you do not need five quarts of oil to run smoothly!

Detox your liver with green vegetables, lemon and these herbs: yucca liquid extract, grape seed extract, artichoke extract, dandelion, milk thistle, barberry, oregon grape root and bilberry. These herbs and foods help to detox the fats and toxic chemical oils out of the liver and gall bladder, thus improving your vision.

All oils are concentrated fat, and they can easily congest your liver and gall bladder, causing slow bile flow, which can cause weak fuzzy vision. When bile acids flow properly, digestion, absorption, assimilation and elimination of food operates smoothly and effortlessly. You keep your liver and gall bladder clear of congestion by eating lots of green foods and eye supplements listed in this book in Chapters **7,** 11 and 12.

Make a valiant attempt to discontinue the use of these devitalized foodless foods, toxic oils and their products. Your eyes will thank you for it with improved vision. And your energy will zoom like never before! Too much oil in the diet, even organic olive oil has been found to slow down blood flow in the arteries. Use all oils in small amounts only— 1 to 2 teaspoons daily, if you desire superior health. And avoid all rancid trans-fat oils in processed foods and most commercial restaurants.

 "If we eat wrongly, no doctor can cure us. If we eat rightly, no doctor is needed."
--Victor Rocine

In the **Chapter Seven**, we will discuss the importance of eating the proper foods, herbs, vitamins, supplements for your individual-constitutional body type, using the **Ayurvedic Health System** from India. **(See Appendix D: Health Consultations, incorporating Ayurvedic Body Typing and the Chinese Taoist Five Element Four Pillar's Body Typing System in combination)**, at back of book. Also, (see **Appendix I: 20 Secret Keys to Health and Longevity).** If you want high-level health and energy, and crystal clear vision, turn the page to **Chapter Seven** and read on.

Chapter Seven

A Complete Protocol and Analysis of Nutritional Body Types for Optimum Health and Perfect Eyesight

Ayurvedic Nutritional Body Typing Health System Protocol

The health wisdom from India, known as **Ayurveda = Life Wisdom,** addresses the three Constitutional Body Types, or governing qualities within the body. The **Chinese Five-Element Health System** addresses the five pairs of internal organs, their relationship to each other, the correct five food tastes for each organ, and the condition of each organ system—warm, hot, neutral, cold or cool? We will cover both system thoroughly in a future book. (See **APPENDIX D** for Nutritional Body Typing Consultations using Ayurvedic and Five Element Chinese Four Pillars Systems).

Knowing your individual body type, i.e., what foods, herbs and health protocol you require is vitally important, and a prerequisite to improving health, longevity and attaining perfect eyesight. Do not take this subject lightly. It can make the difference between high-level health and energy, or weakness, fatigue and constant illness.

Each person was given at birth, a specific individual constitution. The three main Body Types are: **Vata**(Air-Ectomorph-Mental-Thin Type), **Pitta**(Fire, Mesomorph-Motive-Muscular Type), and **Kapha**(Water-Endomorph-Vital-Heavy Type.

The **Vata Body Type** internal system operates through the nervous system, colon, bones, and movement. **Vata's are prone to dry, itchy eyes.**

The **Pitta Body Type** internal system operates through the small intestines, digestion, enzymatic and metabolic functions. **Pitta's are prone to hot, inflamed or red eyes.**

The **Kapha Body Type** internal system operates through the respiratory system, lungs, body structure and nutritive hormones. **Kapha's are prone to watery, crusty or expanded eyes.**

Discovering your Personal Body Type is your first step to restore internal balance for good health and perfect eyesight. A person can also be a combination of these main body types, i.e., exhibit symptoms and characteristics of two body types, i.e., Kapha/Pitta, Pitta/Vata, Vata/Pitta and Vata/Kapha In rare circumstances a person can be a combination of all three body types, which means all three humors are in balance.

A Complete Analysis and Protocol for
(Kapha) Water Body Type
(Watery, Crusty, Expanded Eyes)

If you manifest conditions of mucus or watering of the eyes; or your eyes tear, drip and drain; if you discharge a lot of mucous from the nose and mouth, especially during cold weather; if you have colds and flu often; if you have chest and head congestion often, you are a Water Body Type, and you will manifest the following Body Type Characteristics and symptoms.

Characteristics of a Kapha-Water Body Type

Large chest or breasts and stomach; large bones; overweight, strong physique; smooth, cold, thick skin; gain weight easy—hard to lose weight; thick, wavy hair; large forehead; thick eyebrows and eyelashes; large, wide nose; moist, oily lips; white, even teeth; pink, oily gums; wide, thick shoulders; thick, strong arms; big, moist, calm hands; large calves, feet and joints; hard, thick, smooth, pale nails; milky, whitish urine; firm, mucus-filled feces once a day; medium, cool sweat and body odor; moderate to low appetite—can fast easily without hunger; round, deep, low voice; long term memory; calm, sentimental emotions; conservative faith; slow, relaxed body movements; heavy, deep sleep; seldom dreams or has watery, romantic dreams; great endurance; enduring sexual energy--likes children; strong immune system—heals quickly; prone to colds, flu, edema, asthma, bronchitis, pneumonia etc.; slow digestion; Pulse: 60-70--slow, even, steady, swan-like beat; large, round, watery, calm eyes; cold, damp, bloated stomach--heavy feeling; low hunger; dull, heavy pain; low grade fever; swollen, watery, expanded throat; sleepy after eating; anal itch; excess urine, but less frequent. Healthy Kapha-Water Types may only experience these symptoms occasionally or not at all. The healthier you are, the less watery symptoms you will experience. Follow the Protocol suggestions for reducing water, and you will be delighted with the results.

Water Types usually have expanded watery kidneys and liver, which causes myopia or nearsightedness. They have excess mucous and crust in their eyes, especially in the morning. **Drink less water daily,** especially during cold, wet, damp weather. Less water is required when there is high humidity in the air. High humidity actually causes water retention in cells, tissues and eyes. Kapha's need to dry out in a "dry sauna" during damp, high-humidity days. And get some early or late sun on your skin; this also increases vitamin D3 levels in your body for strong bones and a healthy immune system.

Kapha-Water Body Types Need Less Water, Not More!

Just drink enough when you are thirsty. Over-drinking water, juice or other liquids water-logs the body and causes bloating, weight-gain and fatigue. Excess water in the body manifests in Water Body Types as watery crusty eyes, edema and obesity.

The kidneys, bladder and adrenals are weakened by excess liquid intake. This can cause incontinence (weak bladder), poor eyesight, water-logging of the brain, mental confusion, reduction of stomach acids, which results in stomach bloating, water-weight-gain and yin expanded kidneys, with cold hands and feet. Excess water drinking to "flush-out" the body is a fallacy! Precious adrenal (energy hormones) are urinated out when the body is loaded with water. The body is a self-regulating, self-healing natural organism. You need rest, proper sleep, exercise, natural foods and pure oxygen to heal and keep your body healthy. Too much water only weakens the system and causes weak internal organs and illness! Don't fall for the 'half-a-gallon-a-day-water-drinking-delusion, or you will become sadly deluded. Drink when thirsty and stop! There are no health benefits from trying to "force-flush" the kidneys and lymph system. The kidneys, bladder and lymph require the proper balance of food, water, exercise and rest. Over-doing any one of these natural body requirements is the cause of much illness and disease. If you're urinating 6-10 or more times daily, from over-drinking, and getting up at night to urinate, this can easily lead to a weak bladder and kidneys and incontinence. Moderation and balance in diet and habits is the key to good health and improved vision.

The Potato Juice Eye Bath for Watery Eyes

Eyes that water easily, and form crusts overnight can benefit tremendously from a daily three minute Potato Juice Bath. Grate a raw potato and squeeze the juice out through a cheese-cloth or strainer. Squeeze enough juice to fill an eye-cup, about 2-3 teaspoons. Place the eye-cup, filled with potato juice, over each eye and hold it there for three minutes. Try to keep your eye open and the 'cup' held firmly around the eye. Tilt head back or lie down on your back.

Kapha-Water Body Type Foods
Avoid These Foods if You Have Watery Eyes

If you have many of the above characteristics, you are a Water Body Type and prone to Watery eyes. **Kapha-Water Body Types** cut down or avoid the following **watery, damp, moist foods:** excess water intake, fruit, juices, milk, yogurt, soy oil, canola oil, safflower oil, peppermint, wintergreen, spearmint, licorice, zucchini, banana, beef, salt (one-half ounce of salt holds four pounds of water in the body for weeks); sweets, melons, cucumber, tofu, coconut, grapes, dates, figs, tomato Avoid any foods, liquids, supplements or condiments that tend to create water or mucus in your eyes and body. If you are living in a hot dry climate, some of these raw watery foods will be acceptable. Cut down on them in cold, damp wintry weather, and wait for summer to eat them.

Foods That Reduce Water and Mucus for the Water Body Type

Kapha-Water Types need foods that reduce water, dry-up mucus and balance and harmonize your system. For best results, your foods must be **cooked, baked, broiled, steamed or sautéed.'** They will give your body the necessary warmth and dryness to reduce weight and fat. The foods listed below are loaded with vitamins and minerals, and will fire-up your metabolism, control your weight, improve your digestion and strengthen your eyesight. Occasional no-no foods can be eaten if your weight is normal.

Eat light spiced vegetable broth soups and lots of steamed green vegetables daily. Here is your personal list of foods that warm, boost your metabolic fire, dry-up mucus, harmonize, balance your Water Body Type and reduce watery, mucous-filled eyes. Ninety-percent of your food should be baked, sautéed', broiled or cooked, spiced, i.e., grains, green vegetables, light soups are warming, low calorie, and drying. They nourish and reduce fat, mucous and water in your body cells, tissues and brain—allowing your eyes to function at their best--without excess water or mucous. Eat plenty of these drying foods regularly listed in this next paragraph. Eat more raw food in hot weather.

To reduce water and mucous in your eyes and body: eat more dry foods, i.e., baked red potatoes, yams, squash, popcorn, toasted bread, low fat and low salt corn, rice chips, baked casseroles. Avoid melons. Occasional dried apples and berries is ok. Eat blueberries, raspberries, blackberries, cherries. Melons and larger fruit are high in water, which is the main cause of eye mucous and tissue water-logging. Eat smaller fruit.

Fruits for Kapha Body Types: These fruits are good for Kapha's: berries (raspberries, blueberries, blackberries and cherries. You can eat them raw stew thesefruits. Especially avoid: watermelon, cucumbers, strawberries, all melons. Or you can avoid fruit altogether, especially in the winter. Consume more cooked vegetables, lean protein or vegetarian protein source in this book), whole grains, pastas, soups, root

Perfect Eyesight

vegetables and spices in the winter and eat a little more raw salads and fruit in the summer. Grapes are also good for strengthening and cleansing the liver. Eat them during Summer and Fall seasons, but not during Winter.

Many children develop vision problems as a result of excess mucus in the body. To remedy this condition, use one clove of garlic every day, or take one or two Kyolic garlic capsules, especially during late winter and early spring—February through May—a damp, wet and mucus-causing season for Water Body Types.

Just eat "enough" spices to reduce mucous and water. Too many spices in the diet can cause eye inflammation or red eyes in any body type.

Complete Dietary Requirements: Foods, Herbs, Vitamins, Minerals and Supplements for Kapha-Water Body Type

Vegetables: artichoke, arrowroot, asparagus, beets, beet greens, bitter melon, broccoli, Brussels sprouts, burdock, cabbage, carrots, celery, cauliflower, Chinese cabbage, bok-choy, cilantro, corn, collard greens, dandelion greens, eggplant, endive, fennel, anise, potatoes, green beans, green peppers, horseradish, kale, kohlrabi, leeks, lotus root, mushrooms, mustard greens, onions, okra, parsley, pumpkin, parsnips, peas, red pepper, scallions, turnips, spinach, sprouts, Swiss chard, baked squash and sweet potato (yams), cooked tomatoes, watercress, seaweed.

Fruit: apples, apricots, blueberries, cherries, currants, grapefruit, kiwi, papaya, peaches, pineapple, pomegranate, cranberries, prunes, raspberries, blackberries, huckleberries, lemons, limes.

Grains: corn, millet, oats, rice, rye, wheat, sago, spelt, kamut, amaranth, muesli, couscous, quinoa, oat bran, whole grain pasta, rice cakes, dry cereals, basmati rice, wild rice, polenta. Soak all grains, beans, seeds and nuts overnight before using them.

Non-Dairy Substitutes: Plain organic soy yogurt, coconut milk, soy kefir cultured, almond milk, rice milk, hemp milk—all unsweetened.
Sweeteners: raw honey, molasses, rice syrup

Legumes-Beans: These are perfect protein foods for Kapha-Water Body Types: black-eyed peas, lentils, yellow or green split peas, dried green peas, chick peas, kidney beans, lima beans, navy beans, pinto beans.(Eat beans for protein if you are a vegetarian). "Naturade" Company sells an excellent soy-free "Vegetarian Protein Powder." It's made from pea, rice, potato protein etc. You can add it to your soups, dressings and sauces. Rice Protein Powders are good too.

Animal Protein Food Substitutes: Kapha Vegans can eat lentils, split peas, chick peas, fresh green peas, green beans, tempeh, nutritional yeast, rice protein powder, pea protein powders, hemp seeds, hemp powder. For non-Vegans wild caught fish Is your best animal protein, which has omega-3 fatty acids for your brains and arteries.

Seeds: sunflower, sesame, pumpkin, chia, flax. Always soak all seeds, nuts and grains overnight in water. This reduces phytic acids and enzyme inhibitors, which reduces vitamin, mineral absorption, and reduces enzyme production in the body.

Nuts: (Only eat nuts in small quantities, and only if they are soaked in water overnight). They can be dehydrated at low temperatures after soaking, and stored in glass jars for use later. Almonds, cashews, pecans, walnuts, pistachios, filberts, hazelnuts, pine nuts, pumpkin seeds, sunflower seeds and sesame seeds can be used in sauces, soups, casseroles, dips or butters.

Condiments: basil, black pepper, ginger(dry powder), garlic, chili peppers, bay leaf, caraway, chives, cloves, cinnamon, cress, cumin, dill, fennel, mustard, marjoram, parsley, nutmeg, oregano, pumpkin pie spice, rosemary, sage, savory, thyme, tarragon, apple cider vinegar.

Beverages: dry wines, aloe vera gel, apple cider, apple juice, apricot juice, berry juice, black tea (spiced), cherry juice, cranberry juice, grain coffee, Dacopa, mango juice, vegetable juice, peach juice, pomegranate juice, prune juice, rice milk, almond milk. (Consume juices sparingly (dilute by ¾ with water), and mostly during hot weather).

Herbal Teas: alfalfa, blackberry, borage, burdock, catnip, chamomile, chicory, clove, chrysanthemum, cinnamon, corn silk, dandelion, eyebright tea(for all eye conditions),, bilberrry(for nearsightedness and night vision), elder flower, eucalyptus, fennel, fenugreek, juniper berry, oat straw, nettle, orange peel, raspberry, red clover, saffron, sage, sassafras, yerba mate', Good Earth Tea, "Traditionals"—Cinnamon Spice and Vanilla Spice.

Spices: allspice, anise, asafetida, turmeric, poppy seeds, mace, cayenne, neem leaves. (See 'Condiments' for more spices).
 Oils: Flax, sesame, olive, sunflower, ghee.

Food Supplements: bee pollen, honey, royal jelly, spirulina, alfalfa seed tablets, green kamut, spirulina.
Vitamins: A, B, B12, C, D, E, F.
Minerals: sulfur, carbon, hydrogen, chlorine, iron, magnesium, chromium selenium.

Protein: 10-20% daily intake.

Carbohydrates: 70-80% daily intake. (Grains, vegetables).

Fats: 10-15% daily intake.

Exercise: 45-60 minutes daily. Walking, running, biking, low impact weight-bearing aerobic activity, high repetition-low weight resistance barbells, dumbbells or machines, stair climbers, treadmills, mountain climbing, stair climbing, step-ups, dry InfraRed Sauna; yoga deep breathing through your right nostril to speed-up metabolism.

Special Therapies to Reduce Kapha-Water Body Type

- Hot dry heat. Dry saunas are excellent to dry-up water and mucous in your body. Up to 45 minutes, three to 4 times a week. Or live in a dry climate, like Arizona.
- Emetic therapy to clear mucous out of the stomach.
- Diet emphasizing the three water-reducing tastes: pungent, bitter, astringent.
- Dry, deep massage with lotions made up of hot herbs like ginger, mustard oil, onion and asafetida.
- Plenty of vigorous exercise daily.
- Herbal liquid elixirs.
- Breathing exercises that create heat in the body.
- Chi Kung moving and breathing exercises.
- Periodic fasting from food and too much liquid.
- Reduced sleep time. Avoid over-sleeping—it can cause weight gain.

How Much Water Do You Really Need?

In spite of all the media hype to drink more water, "the more the better, to flush toxins out" mentality, there is no need to over-drink water. Lots of pure purified water is good if you are sweating heavily, humidity is low, and you have a natural thirst for water. However, excess water drinking can easily weaken your bladder and kidneys (incontinence), weakens your adrenal glands (too much water actually flushes-out your adrenal hormones with your urine). Urine becomes very light or "water" colored, indicating excess water in the system. Excess water consumption also dilutes your stomach acids, and causes stomach and tissue bloating, and according to Chinese Medicine, bloats-out the colon, and stops the peristaltic action of the colon, thus creating constipation or diarrhea, intermittently. Eating plenty of organic fruits and vegetables, in the proper season, and for your Ayurvedic Body Type, will give you plenty of liquids that are contained in these foods, along with high amounts of natural enzymes, fiber, vitamins, minerals and other intrinsic factors, that flood your cells with "organic natural electrolyte water." This is what your body really needs to meet most of your daily fluid intake. If you have real, true thirst, drink some water or herbal teas on an empty stomach. Avoid drinking with meals, as it dilutes digestive fluids, and can cause bloating and stomach upsets. There is no need to force water, or any other substance into your body, because "they say you need 8 glasses per day." There was never any medical double-blind test conducted to determine how much water humans need. Now, if you eat lots of meat, eggs, white flour, breads, crackers, cookies, cakes, chips, cheese, salt, hot spices, or take drugs, drink alcohol or smoke—and do not eat 80% whole food cooked and raw vegetables, fruits, whole grains, soaked seeds and nuts—your body will cry out for water because it will need it to literally "flush out" and attempt to reduce the acid, toxic foods listed above. The doctor who conducted tests on prison inmates, found that the inmates recovered from many illnesses and got healthier by drinking more water. Why? Because prison foods are all acid and processed "dry" foods, so the extra water he recommended "helped" to "flush out" toxins and hydrate their bodies from all the heat, inflammation and dryness. Had they eaten 80% or more whole foods, vegetables and fruits etc., excess water intake would not be necessary. This doctor recently died of a "water disease"—pneumonia, which is water on the lungs, from over-drinking! Check out all the research and facts before jumping on the bandwagon of some unproven health fad—in this case—"drink half your body weight in ounces of water." If you eat sensibly, you'll drink only when you have a natural thirst, and your water (kidneys/bladder) and fire (heart/small intestines), and digestive fire will keep the balance within your system. Your vision, health, internal organs and energy will sustain you for a long and healthy life.

A Complete Analysis and Protocol for
Vata-Air Body Type
(Dry, Twitching, Itchy and Contracted Eyes)

If you suffer from problems manifested by dryness and tremors (twitching) eyes; dry, dull, flaky skin, thin or underweight body, dry hair; dry cough; if you have constant digestive problems, you are a **Air or (Air/Fire combination) Body Type** as follows:

Characteristics of a Vata-Air Body Type

Small, narrow shoulders and sunken chest; thin, dry, rough, jittery, nervous hands; dry feet; cracking joints; dry, brittle, thin, rough, discolored, nails and deep ridges in the nails; dry, hard, scant bowel movements; gas, painful constipation; inconsistent, irregular or no appetite for days; low, frail, rasping voice; fast, shifting, rambling, weak voice; changeable, fast, uncertain, indecisive and easily excitable; poor memory; hyperactive, accident prone; ungrounded gait; irregular eating & sleeping patterns; insomnia; weak muscles; tires easily; low immune response; constant fatigue; bone aches, arthritis; spinal abnormalities; schizophrenia (paranoid); paralysis; Parkinson's disease; rheumatism; ear ringing; fissures of anus, nipple; tics, tremors, twitches; heart palpitations; congenital giantess or dwarfism; bow-legged or knock-kneed; impatient, restless; vacillation and indecisiveness; poor self-image; intolerance to cold weather and cold drinks; undue dependence on others; enthusiasm followed by depression; weak digestion; pulse: 80 or over--narrow and slithery; restless nature; dry mouth, throat; fearful, apathetic, loner. Vata problems are compounded if they have Pitta heat within them, along with the airy-Vata characteristics.

Vata-Air Body Type
Avoid These Foods if You Have Dry Eyes

If you have many of the above characteristics, you are a **Air Body Type** and prone to

Perfect Eyesight

dry eyes. Dry Air-Body Types must avoid the following dry foods: dry toast, breads (unless steamed soft), crackers, chips, corn chips, dried fruits, baked foods, hot condiments, i.e., dry ginger powder, curry, hot peppers, cayenne pepper. Avoid any foods or condiments that tend to create dryness in your system. This is especially true if you are a **Pitta/Vata Dual Body Type**, in which case you may exhibit heat or fire symptoms (Pitta) with Vata dryness, and a thin Vata Body Type. If you exhibit signs of coldness and dampness with a **Vata Body Type**, it is best to avoid cold, damp food, juices, raw food, and fruit, especially in cold weather, or feeling weakness or fatigue.. Eat more dry and warming foods and some spices to balance out your cold damp Vata Body. If you have more **heat** symptoms, you have a predominate **Pitta-Vata**—primary **Pitta**, with **Vata** secondary **Body Type**. If you have more **cold, damp** symptoms, you have a **Vata-Kapha Watery Body Type System**. This means you are a **Vata** with a cold, damp system, like a **Kapha,** but with a smaller body.

Warming, Moisturizing, Grounding Foods to Balance the Vata-Air Body Type

Here is your personal list of foods that moisturize and harmonize your **Vata Body Type:** These foods must be cooked, steamed or sautéed' to give your body the necessary warming moisture, vitamins and minerals, which in turn, boost your hormones, digestion, strength and eyesight. Eat thick soups and natural puddings such as, rice pudding, squash or yam puddings etc.

Eat more soups, steamed and cooked vegetables, grains and beans in cold weather. Eat a little more oils and sour foods such as, soy yogurt, apple cider vinegar, lemons, thick cabbage soups, beets and rice/almond milk in Autumn to counteract the dryness of the season. Reduce oils and fats in hot summer months. Eat a bit more raw fruits and vegetables in hot summer weather. Eat more protein in winter and less in summer. Grapes are excellent for strengthening and cleansing the liver. They help to improve eyesight. Eat them mainly during the Summer and Fall months. They are too cooling to eat during Winter in the North. If you are cold, with gas, bloating and indigestion, stay away from fruit altogether in cold weather. Raw fruits and vegetables, eaten in cold weather, make the stomach cold; this creates a stomach pH over 7.5, much too alkaline and cold to generate heat, digestive juices and overall grounding and warmth. Vata's stomach or Central Energy needs to be warmed with cooked grains, thick soups and root vegetables, or fish, to maintain balance. The stomach is like a pot; it must maintain 100 degree temperature to rot, process and digest food properly. Without stomach heat, Vata's suffer from indigestion, gas, bloating, weight-loss and fatigue. A 100% raw food diet may not be beneficial for thin **Vata Airy Body Types**—raw foods are too light, airy, damp and cold to maintain their weight and health. Vata's need tonic foods/herbs.

Vata-Air Body Types need to eat more sour, sweet and moisturizing foods during October, November, December and January—when the weather has a drying effect on their body and eyes.

Important Note: **Too many dried foods will cause dry eyes. Choose your foods wisely and 'see' your vision improve daily.**

Here is your personal list of foods that warm, moistures, harmonize and **balance your Air Body Type and reduce Dry Itchy Eyes.** Ninety-percent of your food should be steamed, sautéed, broiled or cooked, i.e., grains, root vegetables, soups. Protein for non-vegetarian Vatas': organically raised chicken, turkey or salmon, or goat milk and goat cheese is good. For Vegan or Vegetarian Vatas', eat hemp protein, brown rice protein powder, soaked seeds and nuts, Imported Nutritional Yeast, or yellow flaked Nutritional Yeast, *Vegetarian Protein Powder from Naturade*, fava beans, lima beans, garbanzo beans, tempeh, and chick pea sauce. These are warming, moisturizing and nurturing to build and nourish your hormones, cells, tissues, brain and eyes. Eat plenty of these foods regularly. Bee Pollen, Royal Jelly, Ginseng, Ashwanganda are good too.

Complete Dietary Requirements: Foods, Herbs, Vitamins, Minerals and Supplements for Vata-Air Body Type

Vegetables: Beets, carrots, parsnips, peas, seaweed, sweet potato(yams), pumpkin, onions, green beans, squash(winter), asparagus, occasional greens.
Grains: oats, wheat, rice, spelt and amaranth. Soak all grains, seeds, legumes, nuts.
Legumes: Make soups from these foods: lentils, lima beans, yellow and green split peas, chick peas, black-eyed peas, green peas, navy beans and kidney beans.
Seeds: pumpkin, sesame, sunflower, flax, tahini butter.
Nuts: Almonds, cashews, coconut, pecans, walnuts--all soaked overnight before eating.
Seasonings: Bragg's Liquid Aminos, No Salt Spike, Dr. Bronner's Mineral Seasoning.
Beverages: Almond milk, rice milk, Dacopa or Grain 'coffee,' lemonade, mango juice, peach juice.
Herbal Teas: licorice, orange peel, saffron, sarsaparilla, Good Earth Tea(original), Yogi teas, Chamomile.
Mild Spices: Almond extract, anise, basil, cardamom, cinnamon, coriander, cumin, dill, fennel, marjoram, parsley, poppy seeds, rosemary, savory, tarragon. Oils: sesame, ghee (clarified butter), olive, sunflower, flax.
Food Supplements: Aloe Vera juice internally and externally(a few drops in the eyes morning and night).
Minerals: calcium, copper, iron, zinc, magnesium.
Protein: 25-30% daily intake.
Carbohydrates: grains, vegetables, pasta--50% daily intake.
Fats: 15-20% daily intake
Best Vegetable Oils: olive, sesame, sunflower, flax
Non-Dairy Substitutes: Plain soy yogurt, rice milk, almond milk, hemp milk, coconut milk
Sweeteners: maple syrup, rice syrup, fruit juice diluted, (in warm weather only).
Fruits: apricots, blueberries, cherries, dates, figs, kiwi, lemons, limes, oranges, currants, pineapple, prunes, mangoes, peaches, coconut, apples and apple sauce. Eat fruit mainly in warm summer weather, otherwise you may over-cleanse, lose weight, thin your blood and get cold hands and feet in the winter.
Animal Protein Substitutes: Tempeh, soy yogurt, brown rice protein, pea protein,

nutritional yeast, pinto beans, black beans, aduki beans, mung beans. Soak all seeds, nuts, beans and grains before cooking or dehydrating or making seed/nut milks or sauces. If you are on a transitional diet away from meat, going toward a vegan diet, use wild salmon or fish from Alaska, until you can go total vegan. If you want to eat meat, keep it down to 10 to 15% of your total diet, and purchase only organic raised chicken or turkey or other meat. In the "China Study" Dr. T. Colin Campbell showed that eating over 10%-15% animal foods causes cancer to grow in lab animals.

Exercise: Yoga Stretching, Chi Kung Breathing movements, outdoor walking, light weightlifting—10-20 minutes, 3 times a week

Special Therapies to Increase Moisture and Warmth in Vata-Air Body Types

☯ Oil enema. More oil in diet. Sesame oil on skin.
☯ Massage feet with mustard oil during Fall and Winter to improve eyesight; warms the body; Massage at night before bed to sleep soundly
☯ Small, frequent meals—never over-eat or over-stuff your stomach.
☯ Diet emphasizing the three tastes to increase moisture and warmth in your body: sweet, sour, salty.
☯ Warm moist steam baths or water.
☯ Gentle oil massage.
☯ Herbal teas that warm and strengthen the body: Rosemary tea for Vata eyes and hair, ginseng, ashwangandha, licorice, marshmallow, ginger, cinnamon, Good Earth Tea, Cinnamon Spice, Vanilla Spice.
☯ Soft relaxing music.
☯ Healing, warming and strengthening colors: red, yellow, orange, green, magenta, scarlet.
☯ Knee, ankle, wrist wraps or lifting belt for injured or prolapsed limb or organs
☯ Herbal wines: Dracsha, Restora, Chavranprash and Dashmula are all good for Vata conditions, i.e., nerves, kidneys and eyesight; imparts strength, energy, endurance, rejuvenation.
☯ Soft, gentle movements, i.e., yoga, tai chi, chi kung, walking outdoors in the forest, lake or countryside.
☯ Calm meditation that calms the nervous system.
☯ Yoga alternate nostril breathing, performed slowly and smoothly

A Complete Analysis & Protocol for
Pitta-Fire Body Type
(Hot, Stinging, Red Inflamed Eyes or Conjunctivitis)

Whether you are a watery-eyed Kapha-Water Body Type or a dried-eyed Air-Vata Body Type, you can still suffer from inflamed, red eyes if you eat too many sweets, fats and hot spicy foods, which can easily weaken and congest your liver-eye function.

However, the **Fire Body Type** is more prone to hot, red, inflamed eyes. If you have the following body characteristics, you are a Fire Body Type, and prone to Inflamed eyes: Muscular toned body; red stinging eyes; flushed or red face; acne, freckles and moles; early graying and balding, piercing eyes with red lines; soft, pink, bleeding gums; soft, pink; yellow/red, profuse or burning urine—strong body odor; diarrhea, loose stools; excess, hardy, sharp appetite, but stays thin; sharp, piercing voice; critical, forceful bearing, stubborn; short, clear memory; anger, jealous, edgy emotions; fiery leader; colorful dreams; motivated, driven; strong passions, obsessions; dislikes heat, tends to infections, inflammations, tumors, rashes, fevers, skin disorders; yellow coated tongue; reacts strongly to medicine; pulse (70-80 beats per minute)--strong, jumpy; hot, strong stomach energy, fast digestion; feels burning and heat in chest and head after eating hot, spicy, pungent foods; experiences burning, inflamed throat; emotions can go from extreme joy and laughter to extreme despair and depression.

Pitta-Fire Body Type Foods
Avoid These Foods if You Have Inflamed Red, Stinging Eyes

If you have many of the above characteristics, you are a Fire Body Type and prone to Red Stinging Eyes. **Hot Pitta Fire Body Types** must avoid the following dry foods. Hot spicy and dry foods aggravate Fire Types the most. **Avoid:** garlic, hot peppers, raw onions, cayenne pepper, curry, egg yolk, nuts(unless soaked overnight and small amount; millet, corn, rye, chicken and turkey, lentils, goat milk, wheat, black pepper, cloves, chives, ginger, nutmeg, corn oil, soy oil, canola oil, safflower oil, almond oil, bee pollen, royal jelly

Foods to Cool and Balance the Pitta-Fire Body Type

Here is your personal list of foods that cool, harmonize and balance your Fire Body Type, and **reduce Red Inflamed Eyes**. Fifty to seventy-percent of your food should be raw, i.e., fruits and vegetables contain cooling minerals, vitamins, enzymes, fiber and water to keep your hormones, cells, tissues, brain and eyes cool, and functioning at their best.

June, July, August and September is the fiery hot season for most of the country. In the Southwest United States dry hot weather prevails most of the time, and you will need to consume more cooling, raw and moistening foods and liquids if you live there. Eat the foods grown in your own area and climate, and you can't go too far wrong. If the weather is hot and dry, eat more cooling fruits, vegetables and cooling fresh juice drinks or pure water. Sour and sweet foods are beneficial moistening foods. See your personal **Body Type Food List below.** Grapes are an excellent food for the liver and should be eaten mainly during the summer and fall months. They are too cooling to eat during Northern Winter months. Stay away from hot, dry and pungent foods (spices, garlic, ginger, hot peppers, onions, chips of all kinds etc.), otherwise your body and eyes may become inflamed and overly heated.

Complete Dietary Requirements Foods, Herbs, Vitamins, Minerals and Supplements for
Pitta-Fire Body Type

Fruits: Avocado, blackberries, cantaloupe, sweet apples, apple sauce, soaked currants, grapes, melons, papaya, peaches, pears, persimmons, pomegranates, soaked raisins, rhubarb, raspberries, strawberries, coconut, soaked dates, watermelon, sweet cherries, soaked figs, limes, mangoes, sweet oranges, sweet pineapple, sweet plums, soaked prunes.

Vegetables: arrowroot, artichoke, asparagus, beets, beet greens, bitter melon, broccoli, Brussels sprouts, cabbage, carrots, cauliflower, celery, okra, cilantro, cucumber, dandelion greens, fennel, anise, green beans, kale, Swiss chard, collard greens, lettuce—bib, Boston, romaine, leaf lettuce. Avoid head lettuce—contains very little nutritional value; olives, mushrooms, Chinese cabbage, book choy, endive, radish, parsley, peas, rutabaga, tomatoes, turnips, watercress, squash, sweet potato.

Grains: barley, buckwheat, oats, rice, spelt, oat bran, sago, tapioca, amaranth, kamut. (Soak all grains, legumes, nuts overnight before using them).

Dairy Substitutes: Rice Milk, seed/nut milks, coconut milk, hemp milk, almond milk, nuts milks, organic soy yogurt(plain), coconut milk. Get these unsweetened.

Sweeteners: barley malt, fruit juice, rice syrup.

Legumes: aduki beans, black beans, black-eyed peas, green peas, lima beans, mung beans and sprouts, navy beans, chick peas, kidney beans, pinto beans.

Vegan Proteins: Hemp seeds/powder, sunflower seeds, pumpkin seeds, mung beans, black beans, pinto beans, rice protein powder, peas, pea powder, soy yogurt (plain).

Seeds/Nuts: pumpkin, sunflower, sesame, cashews, walnuts, almonds

Condiments: coriander, seaweed (hijiki, kombu), basil, cress, dill, marjoram, peppermint, spearmint, wintergreen, miso, parsley, gray/ moist sea salt, savory, tarragon, thyme.

Beverages: Almond milk, aloe vera juice, apple juice, apricot juice, blueberry juice, blackberry juice, black tea, carob drink, cherry juice, grain coffee, grape juice, mango juice, vegetable juice, peach juice, pear juice, pomegranate juice, cranberry juice, prune juice, rice milk, Dacopa (coffee substitute) grain beverage. Dilute juice by ¾ with water.

Herbal teas: alfalfa, barley, burdock, chamomile, (chrysanthemum and honeysuckle are used internally and externally for inflamed eyes), jasmine, hibiscus, Chinese rehmania(raw), lavender, lemon balm, licorice, oat straw, peppermint and red clover.

Oils: sesame, olive, flax, sunflower.

Food Supplements: spirulina, blue green algae, green kamut, green chlorella, alfalfa tablets. Chavranprash with saffron is a good Ayurvedic tonic paste for Pitta conditions.

Vitamins: A, B, B-12, C, K, U, bioflavoinoids,

Minerals: copper, iron, potassium, magnesium.
Protein: 20% daily intake.
Carbohydrates: 60-70% daily intake.
Fats: 15-20% daily intake.
Eat a little more soups, steamed and cooked vegetables, grains and beans in cold weather. Eat oils or dairy more in dry Autumn to counteract the dryness of the season. Eat less oils and fats in hot summer months. Eat more raw fruits and vegetables in hot summer weather. Eat a little more protein in winter and less in summer.

***Important Note for Pitta-Fire Types*: Too many hot spicy foods can cause red inflamed eyes, rashes, eczema and hot blood. Make wise choices of foods for your Fire Body Type, and your vision will improve quickly!**

Exercise: Lots of outdoor activity and oxygen. Swimming, walking, running, sports, mountain climbing, biking, calming Yoga and Chi Kung breathing movements, calming and quiet meditation. Light weightlifting—do not strain or over-train while lifting weights. Non-impact aerobic exercises are also beneficial. Remember not to get too overheated when exercising, as it could raise blood pressure and heart rate.

Special Therapies to Reduce Heat and Inflammation in Pitta-Fire Body Types

☯ Purgation therapy. Use aloe vera, dandelion, senna, yellow dock, cascara sagrada.
☯ The foods emphasizing the four tastes to reduce heat and inflammation in the body are: you need sweet, bitter, astringent, and salty.
☯ Ghee (clarified butter) or use coconut butter if Vegan, internally and applied externally on body.
☯ Avoid excess heat. Apply cool lotions, pastes and oils made from sandalwood, rose petals, aloe vera etc.
☯Use herbal perfumes, sprays and incense to reduce heat: lavender spray, sandalwood, rose, aloe etc.
☯ Practice slow breathing techniques to cool and calm the body.
☯ Exercise during the cool part of the day.
☯ Perform Yoga bending movements that tonify the small intestines.
☯ Healing, cooling and calming colors: blue, purple, turquoise, magenta.
☯ Meditation by lakes, oceans, trees, mountains—brings peace and calmness to mind and body.

Follow these dietary suggestions as best you can. If you fall off the program for a day or a week, get right back on it. After eating the correct foods for your individual body type, you will feel a new surge of energy, power and focus. Your body and mind become balanced and grounded. Study these body typing principles in other books on Ayurveda and Chinese Medicine. When you study, learn and practice this way of eating and living, you will develop intuition and insight. You'll know automatically what foods you require on any given day or hour. You'll know also when to eat, when to fast or cleanse, how much to exercise, rest and sleep. Above all, your health and energy will increase by leaps and bounds. And so will your vision.

Editors Note
Robert Lewanski, aka, R. T. Lewis, is writing an upcoming new book on Nutritional Body Typing from the Chinese Four Pillars Five Element System, combined with the Ayurvedic Body Type System from India. It will go into much more detail for each Body Type System, and give you an overview of what foods, herbs, supplements, yoga and exercises to do. It will cover all aspects of Holistic Health from a Naturopathic and Eastern model of how the body heals, disease prevention, detection of disease symptoms, oriental diagnosis, the yin and yang of herbs, foods, fasting, the false germ theory of disease, the cause of most all diseases, including cancer—toxemia/yeast/fungus, candida—liver and colon detoxification programs, internal food cleansing and food cure protocols, stress as cause of illness, and the mental/physical and spiritual laws of health and nutrition that govern life on earth.

For a complete a Personal Health and Energy Body Typing Consultation, incorporating the combined power of The Chinese Four Pillars Five Element System and Ayurvedic Body Typing System, see Appendix D for more detailed information on Body Typing Evaluations through the phone, mail or email. For up-to-date information, see www.healthforcecenter.com.

Special Note on Chinese Healing Herbs from Shentrition: Shentrition is a potent, comprehensive superfood and adaptogenic herbal formula of 40 power-packed ingredients. It imparts core power or life force to your health and well-being. Chinese adaptogenic herbs bring your energy up when you are down, and reduces excess energy in the body—it balances or adapts to your body's energy needs. Shentrition supports healthy energy and moods, balances stress response, enhances body detox, supports healthy immunity, improves digestion, helps joints/muscles and promotes longevity. **Moreover, adaptogens are loaded with micronutrients (vitamins, minerals, enzymes, phytochemicals, antioxidants, etc.). These powerful herbs support overall well-being and longevity through their ability to enhance LIFE-force, energy, and endurance. Plus, they help support healthy function of the adrenals glands, which are the body's primary mechanism for responding and adapting to stressors. That translates into noticeable support for athletic recovery and balanced recovery from day-to-day stress too. Adaptogens help your body maintain a centered, grounded state, whatever challenges come your way. Shentrition contains 40 powdered herbs and greens. 100% natural ingredients. Vegan. Fiber free, dairy free, soy free, grain free, egg free, caffeine free. No additives. The most powerful food supplement in the world. Order from Dr. Stephen Rogers at: getshen.com. Health and spiritual teachings: shen-life.com. Shen means spirit. Ingredients: shentrition.com. Or call Erica: 866-497-7436. I use this product daily, and encourage you to order a couple month's supply. Tell Erica you read it here.**

In **Chapter 8**, you'll discover and practice **"Three Extraordinary "Ten Minute" Eye Improvement Techniques."** They are easy to perform, fun and relaxing. They help the mind, body and eyes to totally relax, a prerequisite to attain Perfect Eyesight. Turn the page and enter the world of relaxation and calmness.

The Eye – Xerciser
(Gaylord Hauser)

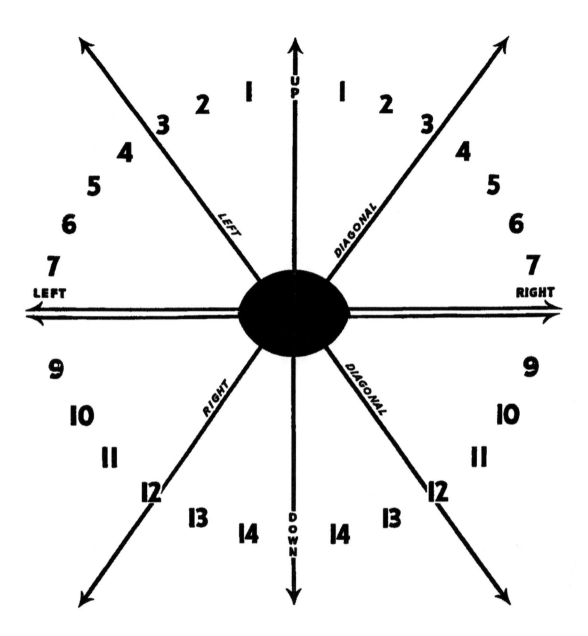

The regular use of the **Eye-Xerciser** will aid in strengthening all of the eye muscles. How to use: Hold Eye-Xerciser 5 inches away from your nose, (or copy this page and tape it on a wall) with nose in direct line with the center spot. Hold your head still and move your eyes on the "up" and "down" arrow 14 times; then let eyes follow the "left" and "right" arrow 14 times. Repeat this process with the "right diagonal" and "left diagonal" arrows 14 times in each direction. Next, make a complete circle to the right, and blink at each number. Next, repeat procedure counterclockwise. Perform entire eye exercise 2 or 3 times per week.

Perfect Eyesight

Chapter Eight

Three Extraordinary "Ten Minute" Eye Improvement Techniques

Sunning, Palming and the Long Swing

These three amazing Ten Minute Eye Improvement Techniques-- **"Sunning," "Palming"** and the **"Long Swing"**—were developed by Dr. William Bates and Margaret Corbett. Dr. Bates based his methods on the principle of relaxation. Margaret Corbett wrote two eye books, "How to Improve Your Eyes" in 1938 and "Help Yourself to Better Sight" in 1949.

Margaret Corbett organized a school of visual education in Los Angeles, California for students and teachers. Many of the teachers she instructed are still teaching today throughout the world. I was instructed in natural eye training by Helen Tolmich for three years. Mrs. Tolmich was a student-teacher under Margaret Corbett. Margaret Corbett's eyesight was so clear when she was past 90 years of age, that she could see the stars during daylight hours.

During the odd moments of the day, practice this short program of **Sunning, Palming** and the **Long Swing**. When you learn to totally relax with these three exceptional mind-eye-body relaxation exercises, you will see dramatic improvement in your vision.

Eye Technique Number One
The "Sunning" Technique

Sunlight is the food of the eyes. Eyes' function only in light. Without the Sun, the earth and all life on it would cease to exist! Mules' kept in a coal mine, without sunshine, go blind in a few days. Many nervous people dread the sunlight, and unwittingly, cover their eyes with dark sunglasses, creating photo-phobia (fear of sunlight). Wearing dark shades does not overcome the fear of light or improve ones' vision. Constant use of sunglasses and hanging out in dark places make the eyes dull and unable to take even the smallest amount of sunlight or brightness.

Bright light makes the eye-pupil smaller. The bad habit of wearing dark sunglasses makes the pupil stay in an enlarged position. Continued use of 'eye shades' over time, actually paralyzes the pupil of the eye. Living indoors all day long does the same thing. The pupil of the eye must become larger in order to 'see' inside or at night. When the pupil is stuck in this enlarged position, the bright daylight seems even brighter to ones' eyes.

Photo-phobia, or light sensitivity can be easily overcome by practicing the **Sunning Technique.** The sun improves the eyes and pupils in many wonderful ways. For instance, it loosens tight muscles. The nerves and muscles just naturally 'let go' of stress and tension, a leading cause of weakened eyesight. Well sunned eyes sparkle and retain their beauty and luster. If you want shinning, magnetic eyes, give up the habit of wearing sun glasses. They deprive the eyes of needed light, weaken eye function and can lead to blindness! The eyes require outdoor light--give plenty of it to them. Millions of sun glasses are sold year around, throughout the world, with no consideration given to their damaging effect upon the eyes.

There are a few good ophthalmologists who are against the use of sunglasses, and are frustrated to do anything about this world-wide 'sunglass epidemic.' Photo-phobia can only be 'cured' or overcome by 'light' itself, eye exercises and good dietary habits.

How to perform the "Sunning Eye Technique": The Sunning Technique is an excellent exercise to relax the eyes and help to overcome the fear of light. 'Sun' your eyes regularly in this manner: Sit down, relax your mind and body; loosen your neck and shoulders. Next, close your eyes and swing your head side to side easily while facing the sun. Turn your head gently toward your left shoulder, then swing it back easily to your right shoulder. Continue this movement and you will soon feel a sense of peace and relaxation.

With practice, you start to notice an 'optical illusion'—the sun itself seems to move to the right as you swing your head to the left and vice versa. Continue this for five minutes and enjoy the warm feeling of the sun bathing your eyes.

Perfect Eyesight

Note: Remember to keep your eyes closed throughout the exercise. After you finish Sunning, 'Palm' for 5 or 10 minutes. The sun feeds the nerves and 'Palming' creates darkness, allowing the eye to **REST.** The sun feeds the nerves, brain and muscles of the eyes. Palming rests and heals the eyes and brain.

On sunless days, use a 150 or 250 watt reflector spotlight bulb. Sit six feet away from the bulb. The sun is a wonderful eye restorer. Make use of this heaven-sent miracle, and experience the miracle of Perfect Eyesight in your life!

Eye Technique Number Two
The "Palming" Technique

After Sunning, 'Palm' for five or ten minutes. Place your 'cupped' palms over your closed eye lids without touching them. Do not place undue pressure on your face. Any pressure on the lids or face stops nerve and blood circulation to the eyes. You want 'free' circulation to your eyes at all times. Also, make sure you can breathe easily and deeply through your nose. Inhale, exhale, relax and "let go" of tension in the eyes, face, forehead, jaws, teeth and neck.

How to perform the "Palming" Technique: Perform the 'Palming Technique' with your elbows on your thighs or on a table. You can also place a cushion under your elbows for both positions. Place palms over eyes. Next, imagine something pleasant and let blackness come into your field of vision. If you see lights and colors, it means you are not totally relaxed—a sign of anxiety and mental activity. You will be relaxed when you can experience and see total blackness while palming. Blackness equals healing, rest and relaxation for the eyes. The positive benefit is improved vision, clarity of mind and sharp focusing eye muscles.

Eye Technique Number Three
The "Long Swing" Technique

The natural holistic health view of disease says: "There is but one disease, toxemia or congestion; there is but one cure, good circulation." Wherever there is a blockage or congestion in the body, energy and healing cannot take place. We need to unblock the blockage, then energy and healing flow with ease, instead of disease. Relaxing the body also relaxes the mind and eyes. A tense body causes tension in the mind and eyes. Illness, toxemia, poor digestion and a toxic, congested colon are prime causes of eye problems.

Dr. Bates and Margaret Corbett emphasized the fact that tension causes congestion— its' cure is relaxation, permitting circulation to flow naturally. Deep relaxation is also the secret of the Taoist Chi Kung exercise movements. Taoist Masters teach us to attain deep relaxation while performing the exercises, thereby, allowing a great surge and inflow of chi (spiritual and physical healing energy) to circulate throughout the body. With healing chi energy flowing smoothly in the body, we can enjoy super health and a tranquil mind.

There are two types of 'relaxation.' One, is the 'Rag Doll Limp' or passive relaxation; the other is known as **'Dynamic Relaxation,"** or exercising, working and moving about while being relaxed.

The **Long Swing Technique,** sometimes called the Elephant Swing, was practiced and taught by the Taoist Chi Kung schools in China for centuries. Dr. Bates discovered the Long Swing in the early 1900s. He discovered that when the Long Swing is performed correctly, the eyesight improved quicker than any other method he taught. This is a **"Dynamic Relaxation Technique."**

In most physical exercises from the west (weightlifting, weight machines, calisthenics etc.), the muscles become tense or tighten up in order to lift the weight. This tightness is the opposite of relaxation. Chi Kung movements like the Long Swing are performed in a relaxed manner. You receive much more benefit from the movement when you are totally relaxed. However, if you do perform weight resistance exercises, never strain or force the weight to move. Exercise without strain, and the muscles build-up naturally, almost without effort. Always finish off your resistance exercise routine with yoga, stretching, the **Long Swing** and other loosening Chi Kung exercises. This is the best of both worlds—toning exercises and relaxation exercises—Yang and Yin (hard and soft). You'll see great improvement in your vision if you follow this program.

How does one relax? First loosen the nerves and muscles, then relax the mind. Shake your arms and legs, roll your neck, relax your jaw, then empty your mind—just put your attention on the movement and breathing. Swinging is one of the easiest ways to relax the mind, body and spirit. Children 'swing' and move their bodies in all different ways. They are happy and have not a care in the world. They are relaxed and flexible--nothing bothers them for very long. We need to become like little children in this respect—not be so uptight and hard in our attitudes.

The **Long Swing** helps to release the energy in the nerves and muscles; it loosens every vertebra in the spinal column; and relaxes the internal organs, thus improving the eyesight, health and energy of the body.

How to perform the Long Swing:
Figure 1-7.
Stand with your feet parallel, about ten inches apart. Shift your weight from one foot to the other, by lifting the heel of each foot as you turn in a swaying motion. As you sway gently from one side to the other let your arms hang loosely and allow them to swing freely as you turn. Move as if you are dancing! Move with an easy rhythm.

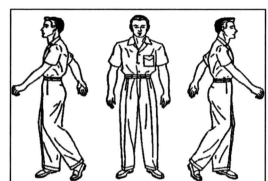

Figure 1-7

Perfect Eyesight

Always remember that your head moves **with** your body, **not** by itself.

Your chest, shoulders, face, legs and neck must be soft and relaxed. Count each swing aloud; this stops you from holding your breath. Never hold your breath during relaxation exercises. Holding the breath causes tension. Easy relaxed breathing is necessary to let go of body tension and mental stress. Perform 60 to 100 swinging movements, one or two sessions a day.

Notice the room 'moving' past you in the opposite direction. When you notice this 'illusion,' the eyes begin to shift naturally. To achieve this illusion, let your eyes allow the room to pass by without becoming fixed to the passing room. Let the room swing by, or as Dr. Bates said, "Let the world go by." Keep your mind on the illusion of the 'moving room.' If your eyes are fixed on an object you'll start to 'stare' and ruin the benefit of this movement. SWING, RELAX and SEE!

This 'swinging illusion' tricks the eyes to loosen and relax, and also breaks the fixed-eye 'staring' habit. This now allows the eyes to shift seventy times per second, a natural occurrence in good healthy eyesight.

Practice the Long Swing for a few minutes before going to bed upon arising, or after 'Palming.' Dr. Bates says: "The Long Swing relieves pain, fatigue, dizziness and other symptoms because the swing brings about relief from the effort of trying to see." It relaxes the entire body-mind-eye complex.

Practice **Sunning, Palming** and **Swinging** regularly. These three relaxing eye exercises are the corner-stone—the basic foundation of your eye-health improvement practice. If you do them often, you'll see and feel the benefits in better health and clear vision. Perform 3 to 5 times a week minimum, 15 minutes each session. You can cure your stress, tension, anxiety, plus improve our vision all at the same time.

The "Black Period" Eye-Gazing Technique
For Sharpening Close and Distant Vision

The **"Black Period" Technique** has been used for years in the Dr. Bates' Eye Training System. We feel that it is a premier technique, along with the **Sunning, Palming and Long Swing Techniques,** to sharpen both *close* and *distant* vision.

How to perform the **"Black Period" Eye Gazing Technique:** Pick out a "Period" in a book from a distance that you can see clearly and sharply. Make sure you have lots of light shining on the page. To improve Close Vision (Farsightedness), place the "Period" **ten inches or less** away from your eyes. To improve Distant Vision (Nearsightedness), place the period **two feet or more** away from your eyes. Gazing at the smallest period you can see will sharpen your vision quicker! Choose a "Period" you can see easily, and gaze at it for 15 seconds—**trace the period** (look inside the "Period" with your eye) and **edge the "Period"** (look around the "edge" of the period.

Perfect Eyesight

This **Black Period Eye Gazing Technique** can be done any time during the day, or during your eye training sessions. This is an excellent exercise for keeping good vision, because it **enables the eyes to focus directly on the macula—the center of eyesight.** Practice with one eye at a time (cover one eye with an eye-patch or your hand, then use both eyes together. Remember to close your eyes for ten seconds after each **"Black Period" Gazing Technique** Session. Relax your eyes and gaze lightly at the "Period." Be consistent with this technique and you'll be delighted with the results.

Do you really want Perfect Eyesight? Turn to **Chapter Nine** and learn the secret formulas that I have discovered to attain perfect eyesight without glasses.

Chapter Nine

Do You Really Want Perfect Eyesight?

Some people think about improving their eyesight, but no one ever improved their vision just by thinking. Thinking and reading about eyesight improvement is merely the first step on the road to Perfect Eyesight. Many like to talk about improving their vision, but you can talk until you're "blue in the face" with zero results. Others' haphazardly practice the exercises. Of course, they receive little or no results. Vision improvement comes only from **regular consistent practice, correctly performed.**

Because of our busy schedules, trying to make a living, raising children or going to school, we have less time for eye exercises. Did you know it only takes about fifteen minutes, three times a week to see results in vision improvement. How much time do you spend in front of the "Brain-Washing-Device" (BWD-TV). Surely, you can find 45 minutes a week to maintain healthy eyes and prevent eye problems in the future. This is my special **'Short Eye Routine.'** If you have more time, perform two eye sessions a week, at least forty minutes each. **Set a regular time for your eye sessions and stick to it!**

Short and Medium Eye Routine for Those with Busy Schedules

The Short Eye Exercise Routine
Fifteen minutes, three times a week

Step 1: Five minutes: Black Dot Exercise.
Step 2: Five minutes: Tai Chi Rocker Exercise.
Step 3: Five minutes: Eye Palming Technique.
Step 4: Lift the Sky Exercise every morning: Six times.
Step 5: Tracking Exercise: Practice at odd moments throughout day.
Step 6: Use your peripheral vision throughout the day, i.e., driving, walking, working.
Step 7: Use your distant vision—look up from your close work regularly.

The Medium Eye Exercise Routine
Forty minutes, two times a week

Step 1: Warm-up exercises: Neck rolls, eye massages; two-three minutes.
Step 2: Black Dot Exercise: Five minutes.
Step 3: Stretch Your Vision Exercise for Myopia: Fifteen minutes, or perform Close Vision Exercises for Fifteen minutes.
Step 4: Tai Chi Rocker Eye Exercise for Close or Distant Vision: Five minutes.
Step 5: Eye Palming Technique: Five minutes.
Step 6: Peripheral Vision Exercise: Five minutes.
Step 7: Chi Kung Exercises: Five Minutes.

Woman Does Eye Routine Only Once a Week and Improves Her Vision Dramatically!

Even with a one-time-a-week eye routine your vision can be improved substantially! Kaye Gowman of Royal Oak, Michigan performs eye exercises only once a week with excellent results. She improved her eyesight from 20-400 (advanced myopia), to better than 20-20 in a few years on this limited eye routine. She really enjoys her eye routine because of the satisfaction of clear sight and the fact she no longer needs the burden of eye glasses or contacts. There is no excuse for not doing eye exercises, because even one eye routine a week can give you good results. Get started! What are you waiting for?

Lady Throws Glasses Away
After Only One Eyesight Training Session

Stephanie Peterson of Ferndale, Michigan was absolutely delighted after just one private eye training session with Robert Zuraw. She wore contacts and glasses to correct her 20/100 vision, before she came to the Eye Training Session. After an hour of performing specific eye exercises, she no longer required eye wear to read or drive her car home. She was totally amazed at the results of just one session of Natural Perfect Eyesight Training. She actually "screamed for joy," as she got into her car.

Perform the Eye Routines with
Fun, Joy and Relaxation

Eye exercises performed mechanically, without focused attention, will not improve your vision. Be in the moment and be aware of each movement. Perfect Eyesight requires total relaxation of the body, mind and eye muscles. Relax the eye muscles, let go of mouth and facial muscles, hands and shoulders. Feel these areas soft and relaxed—let go of hardness and tightness. Eyesight improves more quickly and easily with relaxation and focused attention.

Practice Yoga with a good teacher and learn to feel what it's like to be totally relaxed, grounded and centered. You can also relax with a Shiatsu massage, Tai Yoga Massage, or any type of good deep massage technique.

When both body and eye muscles and tendons are relaxed, vision improves more favorably during vision training exercises.

Avoid 'Squinting' as Much as Possible

Learn to see without muscular effort. The eyes naturally 'squint' in bright light, snow or water reflection. Other than that, squinting to read or see an object only weakens vision. Avoid squinting by consciously relaxing the eye brows. Soften and relax your eyebrows and see without effort. Let outer objects come to your vision with ease. Avoid looking with a hard gaze.

Some people tense the muscles below the brow, just above the eyeball, at the inside of the nose bridge. Myopics develop this bad habit from too much close work. These muscles need to become soft and relaxed in order to see in the distance clearly. Here is an easy exercise to relax the eyebrows...

Arching the Eyebrows

Raise the eyebrows and consciously open the eyes wider, while maintaining a relaxed look. This allows you to see more comfortably and easily into the distance without squinting will not occur, even in bright light or snow reflections.

Perfect Eyesight

Sinus Problems, Dry or Watery Eyes

The sinuses must be cleared for proper circulation to the eyes. Either dry or watery eyes are signs of excessive dryness or water in the organs. The liver, colon or kidneys may not be functioning properly, which may cause dry or watery eyes. The eyes are not "the" cause of eye defects. The eyes only show the effects of what is going on in the internal organs. Pay close attention to your diet. Are you eating too much meat, sugar, fat and oils or dry baked foods; too much water, pop, juice, raw food? Always look for "causes" that create "effects" in the body. Not enough exercise and outdoor activity? Get rid of the cause and the problem vanishes!

***Important Health-Eye Note*: Symptoms of disease, illness or eye defects are only the effects of deeper causes. Find out what is causing these symptomatic effects. Get rid of the causes, and the effects shall not come. The Holy Book says: "The curse causeless, shall not come." "Healthy body, healthy eyes; unhealthy body, unhealthy eyes." Follow the instructions in the diet section and throughout the book to improve your health, which will in turn improve your vision and mental clarity.**

Too Much Close Work Weakens Distant Vision

If you sit in front of a computer, read or perform other close work, be sure to look up from your close work every ten or 20 minutes, for 30-60 seconds. In addition, practice "distant seeing" while walking and driving. Look out the window when performing close indoor work. This reduces eye stress and relaxes the mind and body, thereby improving vision. Also, wear pinhole eye glasses, which can help you focus more clearly on your close work, i.e., computers, reading, sewing etc. **(See Appendix E—Amazing Pinhole Glasses).**

A Stressful Life and its Effect Upon Vision

When problems overwhelm us, we tend *not* to look at objects in the world, but see things as if we are trying to block out life and its problems. As a result, we stop using our focusing muscles; therefore, our vision weakens. A stressful situation that lasts for months or years, is bound to weaken your vision drastically. When you consistently practice the eye exercises and eye habits, your eyes will continue to focus, regardless of how much stress you have. You can handle more stress without it harming your vision, if you know the secrets of Perfect Eyesight as outlined in this book. This is an important point to burn into your memory. Never forget it. The more relaxed you are, the better your vision becomes.

It's only when you 'stop looking' (using your eye focusing muscles), that you lose your eyesight. Then, when your life gets back to a normal relaxed state, it becomes much easier to improve your vision.

Eye Exercises and Moderation: How Much is Enough?

Eye exercises practiced in *moderation* improves vision faster then over-exercising or under-exercising the eyes. Never perform the eye routine if your eyes are sore or aching from the previous eye routine. Let them rest a few days before performing another eye routine. Do not exercise your eyes when you are sleepy, tired, fatigue or when your eyes are red, itchy, watery or inflamed. The greatest cause of poor eyesight is reading when tired, sleepy and fatigued, especially at night before bedtime. The best time to perform your eye routine is when you are full of energy and rested in body and mind. You'll get the best eye improvement results when you are refreshed, energetic and look forward to your next eye routine.

The eyes and body heal during rest periods. That's why I recommend one, two or three days of rest between eye sessions, depending on how quickly your eyes respond after the routine. If you have the energy and vitality to perform eye exercises three times a week, by all means do so. One or two days a week is also good, if you are pressed for time.

Deep undisturbed sleep allows the body to heal your eyes. If you are refreshed and "jump" out of bed after five or six hours of deep sleep, that is all your body needs. If you need eight hours to wake-up refreshed, then make sure you get eight hours of solid, undisturbed sleep. Remember: Fatigue, lethargy, mental confusion, low blood sugar and depression are all precursor symptoms to chronic, degenerative disease, including debilitating eye problems.

Think on the Things You Want

The man who has inspired millions of people in the early1900s–Dr. Frederick Tilney—constantly emphasized that "Action always follows the thoughts you think–so think on the things you want."

Too many people think they are worthless--will never amount to anything in life--can never be happy–feel no one loves them. Is that you talking? It is much better to think that you will be successful, healthy, attain perfect eyesight—reach inner peace and happiness–plus achieve the love you want in a harmonious relationship or marriage.

To achieve all these 'positive' things, we are taught by Dr. Tilney to "burn these positive ideas into your mind." See the beautiful and goodness in people and life. Look for the good in all situations. If you look for goodness, you'll find it. Conversely, if you look for bad only, you'll find that too! Be thankful for your life, your health, your possessions, your family and friends. Take nothing for granted. Be grateful for what you have, and you will get more with less struggle and strain.

If you want inner peace and harmony and love, drop your ego(pride and vanity) that wants to be admired–wants everything to go your way at all costs. Get into the habit of forgiving others–give out words of encouragement and inspiration to yourself and others. We all feel uplifted by an occasional inspirational boost of confidence at the right time from a friend, co-worker or family member.

Depression, moodiness and melancholy are epidemic in the world today. In Chinese Medicine, the liver and gall bladder rule our moods and vision. A congested, toxic liver can cause anger, frustration, depression, and suicidal tendencies. Anger is stored in the gall bladder. A healthy liver instills kindness, calmness and perfect eyesight. If anger is present, kindness disappears. Kindness dispels anger. A clean liver gives us clear discernment, good health and spiritual inspiration. So, start on your liver cleansing program today! Keep the fats, oils and concentrated sugars down in your diet. Eat plenty of green vegetables, root vegetables, seeds, lean protein or vegetarian protein from hemp and peas, and whole grains. You liver will thank you for it.

How to Overcome Discouragement

There is much confusion and negativity in the world today. Over the radio, television, movies and in the newspapers, we hear and see nothing but the evils' of the world. Rarely do we ever hear truthful answers on solving these problems. And when a good answer is given, it is 'knocked down' by the so-called "experts."

If the media doesn't discourage you, your relatives and friends tell you that you will not amount to anything. "It's no use trying to improve your eyesight. It can't be done." "Just wear glasses like everyone else." "It takes too much work to improve your vision..." And on and on. Even your own thoughts tell you "It's impossible, perfect eyesight cannot be achieved." Nothing can ever be accomplished in life with negative attitudes. The ancient sages teach us not to dwell on the negative side of life. Look for the good in everyone and every situation. Be positive in whatever you do. Stop listening to those who discourage you from performing your eye exercises. They will say "You cannot attain perfect eyesight." Instead, in a calm positive manner set out to practice the eye and health teachings in this book. You'll be happier and gain more personal self-confidence when you learn to think and act from a place of freedom and independence.

Each day discover new ways to improve your eyesight. Use your intuition or inner vision to give you answers for improved health and clear eyesight. Superior health and clear vision give you clear insight and intuition about your life, career and future goals. Lighten up your life, and your life will be full of light. Read spiritual, health and positive psychology books to help you understand meditation, energy, the mind, body and spirit. Follow the example of those who have accomplished great spiritual deeds to help the world understand the nature of existence.

The Magic Formula for Success

If there is a "magic formula" for success and happiness, it is the "Thankful Attitude of Mind." Being thankful can lift you out of depression. Success in any endeavor is much easier with a thankful attitude. In fact, thankfulness is considered 'prayer' in the truest sense of the word. If you are thankful all day long, you are in touch with the and Divine Order of the Universe—you are aware, mindful and respectful of others, nature and the Creative Force. You are thankful for your life–your very existence on earth.

Everyone loves to associate with people who are bright, positive, appreciative and thankful. An attitude of self-pity and depression is a curse; it paralyzes your thoughts and actions. Negativity stops you from attaining perfect eyesight and inner happiness.

Begin today to be a positive person. Look for the truth. Be thankful for all the wonderful people and possessions in your life. See the beautiful in everyone and everything. Give yourself words of encouragement. Feel strength, courage and confidence flowing in your life. This is the real "Magic Formula for Success."

Real success is not about money or material possessions or power over others. Real success and fulfillment in life comes from being in harmony with the forces of nature, which is the God Force or Tao–natural spiritual energy flowing through you. Real creative success is being grounded, centered and balanced—inner and outer clarity of mind, body and spirit. It is deep inner contentment and happiness for just being in the moment during your daily work and activities. Every moment is a celebration of your eternal existence. Make your life constructive and creative. Your Divine Purpose, and physical needs will then be achieved, right here on earth

The Empty Mind Technique

Zen, Sufi, Taoist Masters, and Christian Mystics speak about the "Empty Mind." This is a quiet mind–a rested mind, free from anxiety. We continually stress and push ourselves to figure out life and its problems. We eventually exhaust our energy and end-up in suffering, frustration and misery. When you learn to let go of the stress in your mind, body and emotions, and become internally quiet and peaceful, that's when the answers to the riddle of life come to you. Life and existence is no longer a "riddle" when thoughts of how things should be stop. It is in this 'rested' state–an awareness of the **NOW MOMENT**–observing and giving attention to what is right in front of you, that gives true inner peace and happiness. Being anxious about the past or future pushes you further away from doing the things we need to do **RIGHT NOW** in front of you.

If you can "let go" and just watch, your life will unfold in a harmonious manner. The ancients called this true meditation. We can call this "eternal meditation" or "Be Here Now Meditation." You are focused, balanced, centered and grounded between Heaven and Earth. This is also the secret formula to a calm mind and clear, sharp vision. Remember: Vision is a brain-mind (psycho-spiritual) phenomena.

Persian Sufi Mind-Eye Breathing Technique

This Sufi Breathing Technique is known in the mid-East to prevent hair loss, improve vision and overcome wrinkles. It also helps to stimulate and maintain the thyroid and pituitary glands in perfect working order.

How to Perform the Persian Breathing Technique: In standing position, place your feet about shoulder width apart. Close the right nostril with your right thumb and inhale deeply through the left nostril until your chest expands fully. Next, close both nostrils with thumb and forefinger, while bending over from the waist, head lowered, knees slightly bent. Hold your breath in this position for 20 to 40 seconds, or as long as comfortable. While in this lowered position, a strong pulsation of blood will be felt in the head, eyes, mouth, tongue and brain—a flushed feeling from the chest to the top of the head. Next, slowly straighten up, and let the breath flow out from the right nostril.

If you are ill or have high blood pressure, perform this exercise sitting straight up without bending over. If you are in good health, and a little dizziness or lightheadedness is felt during or after this movement, cut back to only 5 or 10 seconds total, of breath holding with head lowered. Build up to 40 seconds over several weeks. However, be persistent, and after a few sessions, the dizziness will disappear, and you'll begin to feel elated and energized.

This breathing exercise is designed to burn up toxins and poisons in the body and purify the blood stream, thus imparting a glowing complexion and clear, sharp vision. Always remember to inhale through the left nostril and exhale through the right. Perform this exercise no more than 3 times per session for its full value, and 3 to 4 times per week, or every day if you want.

The Tranquil Meditation Technique

When your mind is tranquil, mental clarity and vision automatically improves. **How to perform the Tranquil Meditation Technique:** Sit straight in a chair. Relax body and mind totally. Just let go. Close your eyes. Next, simply breathe slowly and calmly in and out through the nose—extend your breath for as long as you can on the exhale, and inhale easily and deeply. Perform this Tranquil Breathing Meditation Technique for 5 or 10 minutes. Visualize tranquility; go beyond your body sensations, and into serene tranquility. If your mind starts drifting and thinking about things, simply place your attention and intention on your breath coming in and out of your nose, until tranquility is attained. It helps to gaze at the tip of your nose while breathing in and out. The mind is focused easier at the single point of attention on the breath coming in and out of the nose. Eventually, a point is reached where your breath becomes almost automatic. Thus, once the breathing technique is initiated and tranquility is reached, the breath or spiritual essence that sustains the physical body takes over. In this state of tranquility, physical and spiritual healings can take place. You are now in touch with the Creative Force of the Universe. Miracles often happen in this tranquil state, including eyesight improvement and disappearance of disease conditions.

There is a couple of authors that I highly recommend for you to read: Nine books by Hua Ching Ni, _Ageless Counsel for Modern Life: Profound Commentaries on the I Ching by an Achieved Taoist Master_, _The Power of Positive Living (Course for Total Health)_, _Self-Reliance and Constructive Change (Course for Spiritual Self-Development)_, _Workbook for Spiritual Development of All People_, _Key to Good Fortune_, _By the Light of the North Star: Cultivating Your Spiritual Life_, _8,000 Years of Wisdom (Book I and II)_,

The Gentle Path of Spiritual Progress: Messages Given by a Buffalo Rider, a Man of Tao. Google Yo San University in Santa Monica, CA, a 4 year accredited, licensed Acupuncture and Traditional Chinese Medicine University founded by Dr. Hua Ching Ni.

And also, go to SevenStar Communications for all of Hua Ching Ni's books on health, spiritual teachings and positive, creative, health and success philosophy.

Plus, read all the books by Dr. Jack Tips, on health, *"Your Liver, Your Lifeline,"* *"The Pro Vita! Plan,"* *"Overcoming Candida"* and more on health. Plus, read his monumental book on manifesting your dreams, *"PASSION PLAY: Manifest your dreams with the 7 minute mirror technique."* Go to Dr. Tips' website for more information on healing, health, herbal bioenergentic Systemic Healing Formulas designed by his mentor Dr. Stu Wheelwright—www.apple-a-daypress.com. Dr. Tips has a wholistic health clinic in Austin, Tx. He does all the latest state-of-the-art tests, with the best bio-devices to evaluate your entire system—glands, endocrine system, hormones, urine, saliva, blood-work, and he outlines a program to balance your whole body and organs.

The teachings of these two authors can bring you back to a healthy positive balance for a life of creative success, spiritual enlightenment, and high level health.

All of the above books can be purchased at www.amazon.com book search at discounted prices. The Perfect Eyesight book can also be purchased at **www.momenntum98.com**, Nutri-Foods Health Store in Royal Oak, MI: 248-541-6820, Nutri Books Distributors: 800-279-2048, or New Leaf Distributors: 800-326-2665, The Tree House Health Store: (248) 473-0624, 22906 Mooney St., Farmington, MI 48336. Also, purchase at www.thepowerhour.com or www.thepowermall.com, **877-817-9829.** Listen to **Joyce Riley**, live streaming at the above website, or shortwave radio (7490 SW)—cutting-edge research worldwide: topics on natural health, healing, world affairs, environment, essential oils, vision, economy, water, new health products—herbs, whole food supplements; new radio guests, authors, documentary producers, doctors, naturopaths and more, every day, from 8am to 11am, EST, m-f. Joyce sells many of the best natural high quality health products in the world. We were interviewed on The Power Hour Radio Talk Show several years ago, and again, soon, when this edition of Perfect Eyesight comes out this year. Stay tuned. And shop at thepowermall.com, and look for frequent discounts and sales specials.

In **Chapter Ten**, you'll learn some amazing secret techniques to improve your vision and to enhance your health and well-being. These "vision secrets" come to us from eye doctors and health specialists from early America, to way back in history from Germany, India, China, Japan and Egypt. Turn the page to **Chapter Ten** and absorb the **"Vision Wisdom from Holistic Health and Natural Eye Specialists,"** past and present.

Perfect Eyesight

Chapter Ten

Vision Wisdom from Holistic Health and Natural Eye Specialists

Eyes Reflect the Health of the Body

The whites of the eyes reflect the condition of internal health. If there is yellow in the eye-whites, liver jaundice is indicated. Constant red eyes reflect a bad liver. A toxic, inflamed liver, according to Chinese Medicine, causes one to become angry, upset, depressed and impatient easily, with reddish eyes.

Professor Chee Soo, a Taoist teacher and writer says: "A gray or blue 'eye-white' color means that the person is losing their eyesight and may, if these symptoms are ignored, eventually go blind." Eye-whites must be clear white.

Purplish-red "eye-whites" could be a sign of color blindness. Black "eye-whites" indicates kidney problems. Green "eye-whites" may indicate cancer; and brown "eye-whites" denotes the presence of stones or cysts. Healthy eyes are clear, steady and sparkling, without red lines or discoloration. A person in good health has very little eye white showing. A very healthy and vibrant person has more iris than eye whites showing.

Clean Out Your Bloodstream and Improve Your Vision

Dr. Benedict Lust, MD., an early nineteen-hundreds' Naturopathic and Medical Doctor states: "If your eyesight was nearly normal in your youth, there is no sensible reason why it should not continue in that condition all through your life. Bad eyesight comes from abuse of the eyes through neglect, strain or the eating of improper foods. All of these causes can be corrected at any time through the utilization of common- sense health methods. The first step is to clean out your bloodstream."

Get Fitted for Weaker Lenses

Dr. Lowell Rehner and Dr. John Ross, natural eye specialists and graduates from the Northern Illinois College of Optometry. Dr. Ross later taught Practical Optometry. They taught natural eyesight training to Army and Navy recruits with great success.

They recommended to, "Never wear glasses while doing the eye training exercises. If your eyes show but a small amount of error, leave glasses off entirely once you start this treatment. If you must wear glasses in order to pursue your everyday life put them on again after each session of exercising, but when, in a week or two your sight has markedly improved, visit your eye doctor and get fitted with weaker lenses.

"It may be necessary, in extremely bad cases to do this several times, over an extended period of time, before your eyes reach their highest point of recovery or until you can dispense with glasses entirely. This however, is infinitely better than changing to stronger and stronger lenses every few years as would otherwise be the case."

The Day Dreamer

"The day-dreamer has the pernicious habit of staring out into empty space, blocking out all vision. They usually hold their breath. They prefer not to see reality; fixing their gaze upon an immovable object, which in turn, fixes the eye muscles and weakens the sight and eye accommodation. This is a bad habit of nearsighted people. Cut out day dreaming! If you must day dream, then close your eyes." -Robert Zuraw

Vision is Your Most Precious Possession

Dr. William H. Bates, a great pioneer in Natural Eye Training says this about perfecting vision: "Vision is the most vital of the five senses. The fullest enjoyment of life comes through the eyes--the color of a flower, the form of beauty, the smile of a friend. At work, at home and at play—most of the things we do lose much of their pleasure without normal vision. You can learn to have good vision throughout life when you learn to use your eyes properly under the conditions modern life imposes upon them."

Comb Your Hair and Improve Your Eyesight!

Yan Shou Shu, a Chinese Health Specialist says, "Frequent combing or brushing the hair can improve vision and dispel bad internal wind or gas. Brushing hair while bent over is helpful for deafness and blurred vision." Try it and see what happens. You might even grow thicker, longer hair.

Distant Vision Exercise:
See Like a Telescope With Your Naked Eye

Edmund Shaftsbury, an early 1900's writer on health and human magnetism, writes about the early American Indians: "The American Indians are known to have the strongest eyes in the world. They have the closest thing to 'telescopic vision.' They can see objects in the far distance that the average person would need a telescope to see.

Here is an exercise that is similar to the ones the Indians practiced for clear, sharp telescopic vision. **How to Perform:** Focus your eyes on the tip of your nose for six seconds. Next, look at a nearby object, then glance twenty feet further, then fifty feet, a hundred feet, a thousand feet, and finish by looking into the horizon. Gently try to see an object as clearly as possible. Repeat this exercise several times for 3-5 minutes, 3 or 4 times a week. Eventually, your vision will become perfectly clear."

Strengthen Your Stomach and
Improve Your Vision

Jethro Kloss, a famous herbalist and author of the classic book **"Back to Eden,"** states: "Eye troubles are caused mainly from a deranged stomach, for they receive their nourishment from the food taken into the stomach, and naturally the eating of unhealthful foods and drinks such as tea, coffee, salt, alcoholic drinks, tobacco etc., weakens the nerves and hinders the free circulation to the eye's. Unhealthful foods and drinks cause impure blood and when the circulation carries impure blood to the eyes, it weakens them. The all important thing is to eat food that will give you a pure blood stream."

How to Prevent Eye Strain and Defective Eyes With the
"Alternate Gaze Technique"

W. L. Woodruff, was a writer, lecturer and Physical Culturist in the 1930s-40s. Mr. Woodruff, who had a full head of hair and sharp eyesight into his 80s, says: "Of course there are several reasons for defective eyes, but the chief cause is **strain** of the fine little muscles which change the focus or size of the pupil (aperture or iris) on the same principle as in a camera. Also, they cause headaches in some cases. While doing tedious work, like accounting or reading, the eye aperture is larger than when looking away at a distance in good light, the aperture changes and becomes smaller.

Now, if you keep the eyes in one focus too long, **STRAIN** results. The remedy is **ALTERNATE YOUR GAZE!** Here is a good habit to follow: when doing tedious close work or reading: Look away into the distance–the farther away the better. Do this every five or ten minutes. Too much tension in any one position can weaken any muscle in the body, especially delicate eye muscles, nerves and tiny blood vessels.

Just try standing in one position too long. It is easier to walk around a long time and benefit the muscles and nervous system because you are alternating the position of the muscles involved.

In reading or other close work for eyes, **alternate the focus** by looking at something distant every couple of minutes or so. This helps rest the little muscles that regulate the eye aperture.

Look Up From Your Close Work

Drs. Ross and Rehner, also place great emphasis on the importance of looking up and away from our close work to avoid eye strain and tension:

"Look up and away from your close work at frequent intervals. No matter how fascinating or important your reading, drawing, or sewing may be, glance away from it for a second or two every few minutes. This is just as important, as it is simple to do.

"If these muscles are kept in a state of contraction for long periods of time without relaxation, they tend to remain cramped when we do finally order them to relax by looking up and away. This is especially true of the muscles of accommodation.

"If you have ever carried a heavy suitcase quite a distance before setting it down, you have noticed how long it takes for your fingers to uncurl. This is because the flexor muscles tend to remain in a state of contraction. The same thing can happen to the accommodative eye muscles when they remain contracted for long periods of time. "By looking up and away from our close work at frequent intervals we can minimize this muscle cramping which causes the eyes to remain focused for near objects when we wish to see farther away."

Discover Dr. Peppard's Secret to Prevent "Nearsightedness"

Dr. Harold M. Peppard wrote "Sight Without Glasses" in 1940. He gives us instructions on how to 'read' properly without straining and weakening our eyes.

"When the print is held too close, myopia (nearsightedness) will be the result."

Step 1: "Sit properly. Spine straight. Hold the head balanced over the body, not bent down or forward from the shoulders.

Step 2: "Hold the book up toward the eyes, not lazily place it in the lap. Fourteen to sixteen inches is the proper distance for reading.

Step 3: "Arrange the light. Have plenty of light without glare.

Step 4: "Read easily and deliberately, word by word. Do not scan and skim. In this fashion, you train your eyes to act normally when they read, and so avoid acquiring abnormal activities.

Step 5: "Read only when you feel able. When you are sick or tired, the eyes too, are tired and weary, and need to rest. Lie down on back, close eyes, breathe in and out from abdomen slowly and quietly for a few minutes. Sleep if your body needs it.

Step 6: "Do not read while eating, or after eating for at least one hour."

Strengthen Your Eye Muscles for Perfect Eyesight

Again, Drs. Ross and Rehner advocate eye muscle exercises to improve eye-focusing power:

"The eye muscles, which have so much to do with the focusing power of the eyes, are the same as other muscles of the body. Disuse weakens them, allows the sight to become stale—proper use strengthens them. Eye muscles needed the variety of "pulls" of diversified focusing intensities. A constant sameness of use is deadening to eye muscles.

"It is only when they are all used properly and enough, that they each exert the amount of pull or pressure on the eye-ball required to keep it functioning correctly so that the light rays come to an exact focus on the retina..." "Also, massage the eye-lids which stimulates fresh blood to and around the eyeballs." Practice the exercises in this book for focusing power.

The "Exhaling Bull" Technique for Eye Power and Rejuvenation

All animals know instinctively the value of exhalation. You have often heard the horse blowing through its nostrils or a dog panting or coughing with vigor. Professor Godfrey Rodrigues says in his book "Key to Life," "What animal has more strength for its size than a bull? When he blows through his nostrils, it reacts like a fountain of force.

The bull knows that the more he exhales, the stronger and more powerful he becomes. Continually "blowing" or exhaling out vigorously, makes your lungs take in more oxygen, which strengthens your lung capacity, and the longer you live. Also, deep breathing in this manner makes your waist tighter and smaller, and more poisonous wastes are eliminated from your lungs."

Here is an excellent exercise given by Dr. George Clements, a Natural Health Doctor and author of many health books, including a complete course in health and healing called "*Orthopathy*", from Health Research Books.

"Exhale to the limit, blowing your breath out as long as possible; increase the exhalation by hard coughing; then hold your breath for a few seconds. This creates a suction in the lungs that draws more poison from the body; finally blow out the last bit of air. In removing the stale air, we make more room for fresh air. After exhaling, the air comes in effortlessly."

Foul air lowers your vitality, while fresh air gives us more vim and vigor. You will notice that after a session of "exhaling," your eyesight will be clearer and sharper. This encourages you to perform it often. You finally get the idea of how important this exhaling technique is for relaxing and rejuvenating your eyes, lungs and health.

To "Blink" or Not to "Blink" that is the Question!

Michio Kushi, the leading exponent of macrobiotics in the world, the founder of the East West Foundation and the Kushi Institute, and author of many books on health and diet, has some interesting things to say about eye-blinking and health: "The standard speed of blinking is three times per minute, or once every twenty seconds. The less blinking the better. Blinking is closing the eyes more, which is a sign of excess yin [water in the body]. "A healthy person's eyes can go without blinking for many minutes; a baby hardly blinks at all. A person who blinks less is currently in a more active sharp condition, in both physical and mental character.

"A person who blinks more than three times per minute is in a state of declining health, due to the consumption of excessive liquid, fruit and sugar.

"If blinking is abnormally frequent, a person is suffering from nervous disorders and is experiencing extreme sensitivity, fear and irritability. If we blink more and more we finally close our eyes and die."

Eye-Blinking Linked to Inner Health, Energy and Personal Magnetism

"We have our best health as babies and young children, provided our parent's diet was good before our birth. Babies are relatively clean and contracted internally. Did you ever notice that babies rarely blink their eyes while awake. Babies also do not show much 'whites' around the iris. Why? Because their cells, tissues, nervous system and brain is not expanded with yin foods: excess water, sugar, fruit, pop, sugars, coffee, alcohol, drugs etc.

"I have observed drug (yin-expansive) addicts and some people on high yin sugary or juice diets (exclusive raw foods: fruit, vegetables, juices, etc.), blinking fifteen to twenty times or more per minute. {In the extreme} they can be high strung, nervous, over-sensitive, super-critical, negative, paranoid and fearful. One can sense an uneasy tension surrounding them. They show a lot of eye-whites, which indicates an expanded nervous system and excess water retention.

"A healthy magnetic man or woman is calm and peaceful. They hardly blink at all. Their face glows and they have magnetic eyes, with very little eye-whites showing. You don't feel nervous or tense around them. They are positive, creative and courageous, without paranoia or fear. They see reality, people and the world with clear insight.

"Excess water or other liquid intake expands the kidneys and bladder, which can lead to water on the brain. The brain, like a camera, records pictures taken in through the eyes. Our eyes are like the aperture of a camera. "Excess water in the body cells and brain causes one to blink involuntarily in an effort to rid the body of excess water (yin). Blinking more does not lubricate the eyes, the eye muscles, eye nerves, or tear duct glands. Excess blinking is the **result** of excess mucous and watery lubrication in the eyes and body tissues.

"When you are healthy, fit, rested, calm and peaceful, you need not worry about blinking–your body will take care of that task for you. A healthy person blinks two or three times a minute. More blinking only shows internal imbalance and poor health. Chinese Natural Medicine teaches us that excess blinking also indicates a weak expanded (yin) liver, a major cause of nearsightedness (myopia).

Observe people in your surroundings. Put this knowledge to the acid test. Watch for signs, symptoms and characteristics in yourself and others. Knowledge without practical experience is useless. Above all, observe yourself. Are you blinking excessively? Are you myopic or farsighted? Is your health below par? Energy low? Fatigue high? Why? Keep digging and answers will be given to you. Knock and the door shall be opened. Ask and you shall receive. After all, it is your own health and vision! Why not do something to improve your health and vision today!

Diet and Dao-Yin:
Health Diagnosis Through the Eyes

Jean Rofidal, writing in DO.IN (Dao-Yin): Eastern Massage and Yoga Techniques draws a close link between the health of the body organs and eye health:

"The eyes have a close connection with the liver and when the liver is functioning badly the eyes ache. When a person has eaten too much or had a meal that is Yin (sweets, alcohol) the eyes are tired and have circles around them and do not bear the light very well.

"The eyes of a person in good health bear everything: blinding light, cold and wind without crying, onions etc. The brilliancy of the eyes depends on what is eaten. A person in good health does not need sunglasses.

"Our eyes betray our thoughts, good or bad, or kindness and our unkindness etc. Frequent blinking (more than three times a minute) is a sign of organic weakness.

"In women the eyes are linked with the ovaries and in men with the testicles. Sexual excess is revealed by black circles around the eyes. In men, the eyes should be small and almond-shaped. In women, they should be bigger and rounder (Yin). "If the kidneys are overworked by too much drink, especially alcohol, the eyes become tired and sensitive, and the puffy lower eyelids form 'bags' under the eyes. A further pouch can form a couple inches under the eyes; bags hang down beside the nose and indicates a degeneration of the intestines. It is often seen in the elderly."

Heed the Warning: Unfermented GMO Soybeans, Soy Oil, Tofu linked to Thyroid Problems, Protruding Eyes, Liver Disease and Weak Immunity

Naboru Muramoto, a leading Macrobiotic teacher and author of "Healing Ourselves" states: "Soybeans are **not** recommended as a bean dish, despite their protein content. [Soybeans are not a building protein–at best they are a low maintenance protein and very difficult to digest].

"The soy protein contains a certain harmful acid which can be eliminated only by elaborate [and long] cooking methods. This is why Orientals usually eat soybeans in the form of tofu, a sort of "soybean cheese." But, to make it less harmful and digestible, tofu must be baked or sautéed until it is hard. This takes out the sticky substance in the fat. Soy products make the blood sticky and weaken liver function, which lowers red blood cell count and depresses the immune system.

"However, tofu is **NOT** desirable either. Protruding eyes [thyroid malfunction] are often a sign of a large consumption of GMO soybeans." This also goes for soy dogs, soy oil, soy burgers and soy margarine, soy powders and soy milk. Organic tempeh, miso, plain soy yogurt and tamari are ok to eat because they are fermented and cultured. Just make sure they are non-GMO and organic.

Obtain your protein from a variety of other beans, peas and legumes. They are easier and quicker to prepare and taste better too, without all the health-damaging side-effects of GMO soy isolates or tvp (texturized vegetable protein).

Ancient Zen-Taoist Technique to Reduce Swollen Eyes

Taoist Master Da Liu wrote in his "Taoist Health Exercise Book": "If Blood circulation is poor, your feet will be cold, since this area is farthest away from the center of the body. A great Confucian scholar believed strongly in rubbing the feet (bottom and top of feet). He proved that swelling of the eyelids could be completely relieved by rubbing the feet every day two hundred times. If you do this exercise every day, it can prevent fever {and inflammation} of the inner organs."

The "Eye-Power-Gaze" Technique

Here is a simple but powerful eye technique that can be performed quickly and easily at any time. O. Everett Hughes, ND, writing in Natural Health Guardian (February, 1958) said:

"I wore glasses for years, but after taking these exercises for a year, optometrists told me I did not need glasses.

How to perform the **"Eye-Power-Gaze Technique"**: Close one eye tight. Put more power to it, trying to shut it tighter. Squeeze the eye hard, while shut. Go easy the first few times. Now change to the other eye and do the same with it. Then with both eyes; look hard at some object straight ahead.

"Look at the object very hard. Put power behind the look. Then look hard to one corner, but keep facing ahead. Just turn the eyes. Put pressure behind that look. Now change and look to the other corner. Remember, don't turn your head. Do this 'hard look' exercise to all corners of the eye. If you notice any soreness, you can put a little more pressure in that direction."

The Secret of the "Steady Eye"

Professor Robert B. Hagmann, a well known natural eye specialist in the early 1950s, gives us his secret to perfect eyesight in the "Steady Eye Technique":

"Understand, our eyes work exactly like a camera; move or jerk the camera and the picture becomes distorted. A moving eye also distorts the vision. We must learn to **hold** our eyes with steadiness.

"During the odd moments of the day, practice keeping your eyes **still**, striving not to move them in the least; relax and breathe naturally. **DO NOT HOLD YOUR BREATH.** Do not frown or make faces; keep the face relaxed; while keeping the eyes as **still as possible**.

"Your eyes may "tear" during this practice; don't be alarmed, just let the tears flow down the cheeks. It's only the eyes shifting back to their normal position. While maintaining the steady gaze, also pay attention to the side areas." [peripheral vision].

A Naturopathic Cure for Weak Eyesight:
"Eye Gymnastics" - Part I

Dr. Benedict Lust, MD., DO., DC., ND., a well-known holistic doctor in the early 1900s, wrote many books and articles on health, diet, eyes and natural healing. This is one of his informative articles on improving weak eyesight:

"To cure poor eyesight means to restore it so that objects are focused right, so that the eyesight is 100% again. In many cases, glasses can be dispensed with and eyes made to see again by correcting the **shape** of the eye ball. This is accomplished in the following way.

"The eye ball is the place of attachment of eight muscles. Muscles which pull the eye up, down, to the side and toward the nose. Like all muscles, these may be either strong or weak. If one or another is stronger than the rest, the muscle will pull the eye ball out of shape.

"Thus, a good proportion of poor eyesight is due to weak eye muscles. The cure lies in making the weak muscles strong and firm again. Eye exercises strengthen the eye muscles safely, and eye gymnastics are a satisfactory and productive treatment.

"The following are simple and efficient eye gymnastics. Perform each exercise twenty times.

Step 1: Roll the eyes "up." Try to look at the top of your head.

Step 2: Roll the eyes down, try to look at your bottom teeth.

Step 3: Look out of the right corner of both eyes. Roll the eyes to the right side.

Step 4: Look out of the left side of the eyes. Roll the eye balls to the left.

Step 5: Roll the eye balls **around,** in a circle; look up, right side, down, left side. Look at every corner, ceiling, and floor of the room you are sitting in, without moving your head.

Step 6: Look at the tip of your nose; make yourself cross-eyed.

Eye Gymnastics - Part II

Tired eyes, in many cases, become congested with blood, due to strain, too much close work or weak eye muscles. Eyes can be **toned up,** blood circulation improved and blood vessels strengthened by practicing these eye care techniques regularly:

Perfect Eyesight

Step 1: Close the eyelids, press the eye balls gently into the socket, hold and count ten. Release. Repeat 10 times.

Step 2: Dip a cloth into cold water. Close eye lids and put the cold compress to the eyes. Repeat.

Step 3: Close eyelids. With tips of fingers, gently placed against skin over eyes, circle the fingers rapidly, barely touching the eyelids. This is a very relaxing eye-beauty treatment."

> **_Important Eye Training Note_: Practice these eye gymnastic exercises two or three times a week for best results. Close your eyes and palm ten minutes after each eye exercise session.**

Oriental Medicine and Eye Health

In an article by Beverly Brough "Who Needs Glasses?" in the East-West Journal/August, 1980, states: "Oriental medicine goes one step further in seeing good vision as part of total health. In the five transformations theory, eyesight falls under the element wood and therefore is connected with the liver, so those foods which affect the liver would also affect vision. Foods that are especially damaging to the liver are chemicals, sugar, alcohol, cold drinks, oily [fatty] food, and general overeating. These foods as well as [too much] fruits and too much liquid cause the eyeball to bulge. When the eyeball is elongated in this manner, nearsightedness results. Farsightedness is caused by a shrinking of the eyeball, due to an excess of meats...[and yang spicy foods].

"One treatment for getting rid of excess liquid in the eyes is to put a few drops of light sesame oil in each eye before bed. Heat the oil almost to a boil, then cool to room temperature and strain through cheesecloth before dropping in the eyes. Sesame oil repels the liquid which is then discharged out of the eye. Splash with warm salt water in the morning. Try this for three nights in a row.

"Another method to free up liquid in the eyes is to grasp first the upper lids between thumb and first finger and vibrate rapidly. Do the same with the lower lids. You will be able to hear the liquid as it is released from around the eye."

Macrobiotic Liver Diagnosis: Your Eyes Monitor the Health of Your Largest Organ

Bill Tims, Macrobiotic teacher, wrote an article entitled "The Liver" in "BODYHEALTH: A Guide to Keeping Your Body Well," an East-West Journal Anthology, 1985:

"For the purpose of diagnosis, we can divide...liver conditions into two main categories: an overly tight and contracted (yang) condition of the liver and an overly swollen (yin) liver condition.

"First we determine which of these two liver conditions is likely to arise due to constitutional or inherited tendencies. In traditional [Chinese] medicine, the liver has been associated with the eyes due to their simultaneous embryological development as well as to their connection via the energy meridians of acupuncture. If the eyes are small or tend to cross, if they are close-set, or if the eyebrows grow closely together or slant upward, there is a constitutional tendency for the liver to develop problems from becoming overly contracted. If the eyes are large of tend to move outward or if the eyes are set far apart, there will be more of a tendency for the liver to become swollen. In addition, any inherited or congenital eye defects will usually indicate some related weakness in the liver.

"...most important in determining the present liver condition, is a thorough assessment of the eyes. If yellow, fatty excess accumulates in the whites of the eyes, this shows a similar fat accumulation in the liver. (This often will ooze or crust {Kapha/Water Body Type}, in the corners of the eyes, particularly during sleep when the liver does most of its cleansing of fats from the blood.) If the eyes are red or bloodshot {Pitta/Fire Body Type} or if a rash or inflammation arises between the eyes, this suggests a swollen and inflamed liver condition. The eyes or eyelids or the area between the eyes also...develop red spots or stys, a sign of excessive storage of animal protein in the liver.

"If the eyes become watery or swollen or begin to burn or itch, this indicates an overly swollen liver. ...dryness {Vata/Air Body Type}, indicates an overly contracted condition. If there appears a single, deep vertical line between the eyes, the liver is overly contracted, [yang-tight] which if there are several shallow vertical lines, the liver is overly expanded [yin-loose]. Crossed eyes, down-turned eyes, and farsightedness all indicate a contracted liver condition; eyes drifting outward and upward as well as nearsightedness, all indicate an expanded liver condition.

"A contracted liver condition is caused by an excessive consumption of meat, eggs, cheese and baked goods, while an expanded liver condition is caused more by an excessive consumption of drugs, stimulants, alcohol,...citrus fruits, refined sugar, vinegar, fats, dairy and oil. "...most people have serious health problems resulting from some combination of these foods. In order to restore balance and revive the liver, ...increase your consumption of whole cereal grains and beans, and...eat fresh an lightly cooked green leafy vegetables."

Special Liver Cleansing and Strengthening Eye Foods

These specific liver and eye foods and herbs are the most powerful for cleansing, healing and strengthening the eyes, liver and gall bladder: **Cabbage, beets, olives,**

mangos, lemons, raspberries, dandelion greens, grapes, lychii berries, tomato, celery, carrots, plums, prunes, apple cider vinegar, pickles, **umebushi plums, miso, limes.** Western and Eastern Herbs that clear away liver toxicity and help improve the eyesight: **Eyebright, chrysanthemum, bilberry, Yucca, dandelion leaf, bupleurum, rose hips, haritaki, amalaki.**

Improve Your Vision by Barefoot Walking in the Water on the Beach or the Grass

World Health Teacher-Educator, Dr. Bernard Jensen, author of many books on colon therapy, Iridology and health rejuvenation, recommends walking in a bed of sand, with cold water up to your ankles. Walking barefoot in the grass is also very effective.

Dr. Jensen says: "Persons with poor circulation in the lower extremities put an extra burden upon the heart. When there is but slight muscular contraction in the lower extremities, blood is not properly returned to the heart, and leg disorders may develop. To remedy this condition, we devised at the sanitarium...the sand walk.

"Every morning we wet down a bed of sand with cold water and patients walk in this cold sand. This massaged the bottoms of their feet and developed the small muscles in their feet and legs. One of the first comments usually made by these patients was that as a result of these sand walks they had warm feet when going to bed at night, whereas never before had they gone to bed with warm feet. The Kneipp grass walk, as used in sanitariums in Germany, is another excellent means of increasing circulation in the lower extremities.

"I have noticed changes in patients using the sand walk or the grass walk that are hard to believe. In most cases the whole body responds when we build strong healthy feet; organs are reflexly released. Eye conditions improve almost immediately. In fact, **I have seen eyes improve to such an extent that glass were no longer needed."** (Emphasis added).

Easy No-Routine Natural Eye Exercises

Easy Distant Vision Strengthening Exercises:
☯ Focus your vision on a bird in flight
☯Focus your vision on a moving ball or object at sporting events
☯ Practice juggling a ball
☯ Gaze at a moving car until it is out of sight
☯ Practice 'Distant Seeing'--"trace" distant objects, i.e., car, tree, house, letters, signs, etc.
☯Gaze as far as you can see into the horizon, or at the night stars
☯ For relaxation: Look at nature's bounty--trees, flowers, lakes, oceans, grass, etc.
☯ Gaze at the night moon. Look at the 'red' rising or setting Sun

Perfect Eyesight

Easy Exercises to Boost "Close Vision"
- Gaze at a tiny period for 20 seconds
- Look up from your close work (reading, writing, computers) every few minutes
- Perform the "Eye Palming Technique" often throughout the day
- Close eyes often and relax your mind and thoughts
- "Trace" close objects or letters 20 inches or less away from you.

Easy "Peripheral Vision" Strengthening Exercises
- When walking or traveling in your car, notice the surrounding objects moving toward you and past you. While looking **straight ahead** observe objects to your left, right, up and down. Do not move your eyes. See "objects" with your "peripheral vision only.

Easy "Natural Pupil" Strengthening Exercise
- Go outside; cover your eyes for 2 seconds; next, uncover your eyes for 2 seconds.
- Keep your eyes open throughout this entire "Pupil Exercise." Perform this exercise for one or two minutes
- Sit next to a light switch; next, turn light on for 1 second; next, turn light off for 3 or 4 seconds. Perform this exercise for 2 minutes

How to Improve Distant Vision Using "Positive Lens" Glasses

A few eye doctors, in the early 1900s gave their clients "positive lens" glasses to help overcome nearsightedness (myopia). The nearsighted clients who had 20/100 vision or less obtained excellent results with the use of "positive lens" eye glasses. These "positive lens" glasses are usually given to those who have weak close vision. But in this case, these glasses are given to help nearsighted people see better in the distance. Here's a short explanation of how to use the "Positive Lens" glasses.

Go to a K-Mart or Dollar Saver Store and purchase three pairs of "positive lens" glasses of different strengths as follows. Look on the eye glass lens for a number, which indicates its strength, thusly--+1.00, +2.00 and +3.00. These glasses sell for only a few dollars in most discount stores.

How to use the "Positive Lens" glasses

Step 1: Begin by using the +1.00 lens glasses. Sit in outdoor or bright indoor lighting. Hold printed page in front of your eyes, and move it to a distance where you can see it clearly.

Step 2: Trace a letter on the page with your eyes; next, close eyes for ten seconds and relax.

Perfect Eyesight

Step 3: Open your eyes while inhaling a gentle breath and gaze at the same letter.

Step 4: Move print one inch further away from your eyes and repeat the above steps.

Step 5: Continue to move the print further away in 'one inch' increments, as long as you are able to still read the 'letter.' If print becomes too blurry, move printed page back to where you can read it without strain.

Do not be in a hurry to improve your vision with this exercise. Make sure you can see the letter clearly before moving the print another inch away from your eyes. For example, if your distance in only 11 inches away from the print. Stay with this distance until the print becomes clear, then move it to 12 inches.

The ultimate goal of this exercise (using +1.00 lens glasses) is to be able to read the print clearly at least 20 inches away from your eyes. After you succeed with this 'lens,' change to your +2.00 lens glasses. And finally, when you can see the print 20 inches with the +2.00 lens, change to the +3.00 lens glasses and work your way to the 20 inch mark.

When using the +3.00 lens glasses, and you can easily see the printed page at 12 inches away from your eyes, you will have obtained 20-20 vision. At 20 inches away with the +3.00 lens glasses, you'll be seeing much better than 20/20.

Practice this exercise two to three times per week, for 15 minutes each session. Finish your session by "Palming" your eyes for five minutes. Do not over-exercise your eyes. Vision improves faster when eye exercises are performed moderately. When performing this technique with other nearsighted exercises in this book, do not go over one hour per eye session total. Use your good judgment on the exercises that best fit your eye condition.

"The Myopia Myth" by Donald S. Rehm explains how to use 'positive lenses' in the treatment of nearsightedness. It is published by the Internatinoal Myopia Prevention Association, R.D. 5, Box 171, Ligonier, PA 15658.

The Art Of Reading
Wm. H. Bates, M. D.

When reading, you should look at the white spaces between the lines and not directly at the lines themselves. The reason for this is that it is no effort to sweep the eyes over a plain background. Fixing the eyes on individual words and letters involves strain, and strain impairs vision. When a person with normal sight regards the white spaces with a sweeping shift across the page from margin to margin, he can read easily, rapidly and without fatigue.

If the same person looks at the letters, the eyes grow tired and the vision becomes poor.

People who cannot read well at the near point always tend to fix their attention on the print. Consequently they see worse. Improvement cannot take place until they learn to look at the white spaces between the lines. Reading can be improved by improving the power to remember or imagine whiteness. This improvement can be achieved in the following way. Close your eyes and imagine something even whiter than the page before you--white snow, white starch, white linen. Then open your eyes again. If your mental images of whiteness have been clear and intense, you will find that the white spaces between the lines will appear for a few moments to be whiter than they really are. Repeat this process as a regular drill. When your imagination of whiteness has become so good that you can constantly see the spaces between lines as whiter than they really are, the print Will seem bleaker by contrast and the eye will find itself reading easily and without effort or fatigue.

The Thin White Line

When the imagination of whiteness has reached its maximum intensity, it often happens that one can see a thin white line much better than the rest of the white space. This white line may be compared to a neon light moving swiftly from one margin to the other immediately under the letters.

Consciousness of this thin white line is a great help in reading, increasing as it does the speed both of the eyes and of the mind. Once this illusion of the white line is seen, imagined or remembered, unlimited reading without fatigue becomes possible.

Ayurvedic "Nasal Wash" for Clear Vision

Ayurvedic Medicine from India has taught for thousands of years the importance of cleansing the nasal passage-ways to clear the sinius cavities and to attain 20/20 clear vision and beyond! They recommend using a *Neti Pot*, a little ceramic pot, that holds about 10 to 12 ounces of water. The *Neti Pot* has a three inch slender nozzle attached to one end to insert into the nose. The *Neti Pot* is unsurpassed in cleansing the entire sinus cavity, which helps to clear up sinus congestion, colds, mucous, which can all create poor vision. Frequent use of the *Neti Pot* can help your vision stay clear and sharp.

Swami Devi Dayal of India, from his Ashram Center, has this to say about the healing effects of the Nasal Wash:

"The Nasal Wash helps to relieve nasal congestion in a few days or weeks. Pyorrhea can be cured in a month or two. Hearing and eyesight are greatly improved in three months. It helps stammering in two months. It strengthens the nerves, clears pimples. Memory is improved. One sleeps deeper and sounder. Snoring is diminished. Migraine headaches are relieved. Mental problems helped. It also helps to prevent and overcome TB, asthma, fevers etc.

How to perform the *Neti Pot* Nasal Wash: Fill a Neti Pot (which can be purchased at a health food store) with purified lukewarm water and add about 1/4 teaspoon of sea salt. Next, tilt your head down low over a sink to the right (face is pointing toward your left shoulder) and insert the *Neti Pot* nozzle into your left nostril. Let the water pour into the left nostril *slowly*. The water pours out of the right nostril. Repeat the same procedure with the opposite nostril over the sink.

Next, tilt your head backward and let the water flow up your right nostril so it runs into your mouth; then spit it out. With your head in this backward position, close the opposite nostril with your finger, so the water will go into the mouth. Repeat with the left nostril. It is recommended to practice the **Neti Pot Nasal Wash** daily for a few weeks, for optimum health benefits. Here is some deep wisdom from the Yoga Ratnakara, a treatise on Ayurvedic Medicine: "A person who regularly drinks water through the nose in the early morning and at night, becomes intelligent, develops eyesight as acute as an eagle, prevents graying hair, and wrinkling of skin, and is freed from all diseases."

This is a powerful statement indeed! However, Yogis who practice the Nasal Wash Technique, along with other physical, health and spiritual disciplines, are known for their superb health, tranquility and longevity. One never knows until they try it. Give it a try for a few weeks, and find out for yourself if you can avoid those nagging colds, sinus, brain fog and eye problems.

]

Chinese Taoist Secret Longevity Eye Exercise

This is a secret eye technique taught by long lived Taoist Masters from the mountains of China. These sages never lose their vision and they are reportedly over one hundred years young and as spry as spring chickens! Master Da Liu, a Tai Chi Master from China, lived to 100, and taught these practices to his many students in New York City for 30 years.

How to perform the Taoist Longevity Eye Exercise: Sit up with your back straight. Close your eyes. With your first two finger pads, press lightly on the closed eyelids:

Step 1. Inhale gently, hold your breath and move your eyes three times up and down. Exhale. Take a deep breath and relax. Repeat again.

Step 2. Inhale gently. Hold your breath, and move eyes three times sideways. Exhale. Take a deep breath and relax. Repeat again.

Step 3. Inhale gently. Hold your breath. Move eyes in a clockwise direction three times. Exhale. Take a deep breath and relax. Repeat again.

Step 4. Inhale gently. Hold your breath. Move eyes in a counter-clockwise direction three times. Exhale. Take a deep breath and relax. Repeat again.

While performing the eye movement, gently press your fingers on your closed eyelids. The value of this special eye exercise lies in combining **massage** (pressing the closed eyelids with your fingers), **deep breathing,** and **eye exercise movement** simultaneously. You can also press your palm on the closed eyelids while performing this technique.

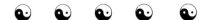

Natural Ways to Perfect Eyesight Outline

Dr. Alexis Carroll from the Rockerfeller Medical Institute, in the 1930s, wrote a classic book entitled "Man the Unknown." Dr. Carroll kept a chicken heart alive for 20 years in a Petri dish by following this procedure:

1. Proper Nutrition; 2. Proper Elimination, and; 3. Good Circulation or exercise. We can improve our own vision and health by following the same example as Dr. Carroll in this manner:

1. Nourish the eyes with nutrient dense organic foods, supplements, herbs.
2. Clear toxins from the eyes, liver, stomach and colon by periodic cleansing diets or elimination fasts, and eating properly, and following good health habits.
3. Strengthen the eye muscles with specific eye improvement exercises, as outlined in this book.

1. Methods of Cleansing the Eyes of Toxins

a. Cleanse the Liver with an elimination detox diet or "fasting," on fruits and vegetables, vegetable juices, dandelion root, eyebright, Lutein, barberry, bilberry, milk thistle, bupleurum, chrysanthemum and other herbal teas,
b. Hot and cold(hydrotherapy) cloth over eyes, or use eye cup
c. Eye drops or eye wash (lemon, apple cider vinegar, cayenne in water.
d. Stop junk foods, trans fats, margarine, aspartame, sucralose, sugar, white flour, white rice, commercial dairy, fast food
e. Nasal douche. Nasal massage with finger and lavender oil
f. Yoga Headstand (3 minutes), or slant board
g. Healing Sound for Liver: Sssshhhhh; visualize the color green and kindness while inhaling, and exhale anger and unkindness
h. Exercise overall body 3-4 times per week for circulation, "happy brain endorphins," nerve health, elimination, liver detox. Walk outdoors 1 to 2 miles per day.

2. Feed the Eyes

(Help for Diabetic Retinopathy & Age related Macular Degeneration). Refer to: *Alternative & Complementary Therapies* Magazine April 2002 Vol. 8, no. 2 (914-834-3100)

a. Organic foods, super food supplements, spirulina, alfalfa, chlorella, blue green algae, nutritional yeast, acidophilis, Gingko 160mg, coQ10(50-150mg divided doses, Vitamin E 400-800, Vit. A(fish oil)10,000 IU, or Black Currant Seed oil for Omega 3 Essential Fatty Acids, Lutein 10-20mg, Quercetin(400mg 4xday, Selenium 200 mcg, Rutin 1.000, Alpha Lipoic acid 500-900 mg, Magnesium 350mg, Bioflavanoids 1,000mg, Bilberry 200-480mg, Melatonin 200 mcg. 2-3 hours before bed
b. Milk Thistle, 2-4 capsules daily
c. Eye Sunning feeds the eyes
d. Eat only when hungry, don't overeat
e. Drink only when thirsty—don't over-drink any liquids

3. Strengthening the Eye Muscles with Eye Exercises

a. Focus on close and distant objects exercises focusing muscles
b. Strengthening the ciliary muscles, so light can focus directly on macula for vision
c. Stretch your eyes (up/down, side to side, diagonal. Turning muscles
d. Strengthen Pupils: lights on & off, stand in shade and sun
e. Squeezing muscles—squeeze eyes tight (muscles that close eyes)
f. Open eyes wide—breathe out liver "ssshhh" sound with eyes wide open
g. Look close, then look far. Strengthens Accommodating muscles (follow bird, baseball, car license plate—let eyes follow object as far as it can see it
h. Most people over 50 lose ability to Accommodate (look close and far)

i. Obtain plenty of sleep, rest, especially when tired, stressed or exhausted
j. Perform eye palming at least 5 minutes daily.

Natural Eye Focusing Exercise

Place your eye chart on the wall with good light shining on it.

Perform this Eye Focusing Exercise at least 3 times per week.

This is the primary exercise that allows all the other eye exercises to work correctly.

Step 1. Stand 6 to 12 inches away from the eye chart letters.

Step 2. Gaze at the smallest line you can see and read.

Step 3. Trace each letter on the line you can see.

Step 4. Close your eyes for 15 seconds, and relax facial and eye muscles.

Step 5. Open eyes and look at the letters again.

Step 6. Palm your eyes for 15 seconds.

Step 7. Open eyes and look at the letters on the Eye Chart again.

Next, move one more foot away from Chart and perform the same steps as above. Next, move another foot away, and keep moving back one foot at a time, away from the Eye Chart until you reach five feet away. As you move back away from the Eye Chart, always choose the smallest line you can actually read, while Tracing, closing the eyes and palming. Strive to see these letters more sharply and clearly. If you relax properly, the letters will come in, more clearly.

You can use this same technique for the Tibetan Eye Chart and the Black Dot Eye Exercises. With your eyes Trace or color-in the Tibetan Eye Chart; next close your eyes for 15 seconds; next, open your eyes and look at the Chart; next, palm or cup your hands over your eyes for 15 to 30 seconds; next, open your eyes and look at the Tibetan Chart again. Move back another foot, and repeat this sequence. Do the same for the Black Dot Exercise. Choose a Black Dot that you can see fairly clearly, and repeat the entire sequence as the above Tibetan Eye Chart Exercise.

These Eye Focusing Exercises help you improve your close and far vision, by strengthening the eye focusing muscles, which enable you to see clearly.

Five Minute Eye Chart Exercise Routine

1. Look at eye chart 24 inches away--any line you can see clearly.
2. Trace** and Edge* each letter of the line you can read clearly.
3. Close your eyes for 10 seconds.
4. Next, take a deep breath
5. Open eyes and look at the same line again.
6. Palms over eyes for 20 seconds (Palming method)
7. Take a deep breath
8. Look at the line and see if you can read it, or go a line down lower if you can.
9. Repeat this sequence 4 times per session
10. Perform this exercise at least 3 or 4 times a week or more if you want.

*Edging is going around the outside and inside of a letter in all its details.

**Tracing is looking at the whole letter, or going over the letter like you are tracing or coloring it on a paper.

If one eye is stronger, put an eye patch on the stronger and go through this routine looking only with the weak eye, with the eye patch on the strong eye. Just play with it and you will be delighted with the results.

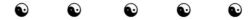

This is the end of the main teachings on vision and eye training techniques and practices. The rest of the book will focus on the latest clinical discoveries on supplements, herbs, foods to help macular degeneration, cataracts, glaucoma and other eye problems.

We hope you have enjoyed reading these **Perfect Eyesight** training techniques and secrets as much as we enjoyed writing it. We challenge you now to take the next step in your quest for improved vision. That next step is practical application: **Practice, Persistence** and **Consistency!** Others' have perfected their eyes, and so can you. Start on your eye training program today and enjoy the blessings of **Perfect Eyesight** for the rest of your long healthy life! (See **Appendix C** on Earthing/Grounding for healing and vision improvement. See earthinginstitute.net for Earthing book and Grounding products. Also, google or youtube "Longevity Now Conference," and David Wolfe. Many videos.

Chapters **Eleven** and **Twelve** cover some very fascinating research and discoveries in helping improve degenerative eye conditions, from major University studies and double-blind clinical trials, from around the world. This is the absolute latest up to date findings, by medical researchers on eye and vision supplements, vitamins, minerals, herbs and foods. First, we start with **"Cataract Studies from an Internet Website"** next……

Cataract Studies from an Internet Website That May Help to Improve Your Vision

http://www.i-care.net/eyeresearch.html/#cataract

1. Subjects taking vitamin C supplements for more than 10 years had a 45-77% lower risk of early lens opacities (cataracts) and 83% lower risk of moderate lens opacities. The higher the serum levels, the lower the risk of cataracts. Jacques, et al. The American Journal of Clinical Nutrition, Oct. 1997. S.E. Hankinson, et al. 1992. BMJ: 305: 335-339. Simon JA, Hudes ES J Clin Epidemiol 1999 Dec;52(12):1207-11

2. Vitamin E, vitamin C, alpha-lipoic acid, and taurine appear to offer protection against lens damage caused by low level radiation. Bantseev, et al. Biochem Mol Biol Int 1997 Sep;42(6):1189-97.

3. Dietary lutein and cryptoxanthin were associated with 70% lower risk of nuclear cataracts in those under age 65. Lyle, et al. Am J Clin Nutr 1999 Feb;69(2):272-7.

4. Dietary intake of protein, vitamins A, C, E, and carotene, niacin, riboflavin, and thiamine significantly decreased the risk of all cataract types. (Combining a variety of antioxidant nutrients produced the greatest effect.) Cumming RG, et al. Ophthalmology 2000 Mar;107(3):450-6 Leske, et al Arch Ophthalmol 1991 Feb;109(2):244-51.

5. Vitamin E taken with bilberry extract stopped the progression of senile cortical cataracts in 97% of the eyes of human subjects. Ann Ottalmol Clin Ocul, 1989.

6. Low blood levels of vitamin E were associated with approximately twice the risk of both cortical and nuclear cataracts, compared to median or high levels. Vitale, et al. Epidemiology 1993 May;4(3):195-203

7. Smokers were 2.6 times as likely to develop posterior subcapsular cataracts than nonsmokers. Hankinson, et al. JAMA 1992 Aug 26;268(8):994-8

8. Patients with senile cataracts were found to have significantly lower blood and intraocular levels of the mineral selenium than controls. Karakucuk S, et al. Acta Ophthalmol Scand 1995 Aug;73(4):329-32

9. Alpha lipoic acid can help prevent cataract formation as well as nerve degeneration and radiation injury. Packer, et al. Free Radic Biol Med 1995 Aug;19(2):227-50

Chapter Eleven

Protecting and Preserving Clear Vision and Healthy Eyes

Help for Cataracts, Glaucoma and Macular Degeneration Plus, Powerful Eye Supplement Protocol for All Degenerative Eye Conditions

No one wants to go blind. The elderly fear that the most because they develop high incidences of cataract, glaucoma and macular degeneration.

Here is good news for you: degenerative eye disease is not inevitable. Scientific studies positively show that eye diseases via lifestyle and nutritional modifications can be reversed and prevented. Many eye degenerative eye problems are preventable. Cataract operations are on the rise to the tune of 3.5 billion dollars a year. Cataract surgery is easily performed with a simple procedure. Complications can occur, and if all goes well, recovery is rapid. The surgery is complex and delicate. On the other hand, problems can crop up during and after surgery. Complication rates can vary significantly from surgeon to surgeon.

Complication rates on eye surgery are considered low, a small fraction of 1.3 million surgeries results in a significant number of people (about 26,000 to 28,000 people in the U.S.) being affected. Some eye surgeries develop secondary glaucoma, detached retinas, corneal edema, eye infections (which can result in the complete loss of the eye.

Twenty to thirty percent of cataract surgery develop (clouding) of the lens capsule. This capsule was originally part of the patient's own lens but was left in the eye to hold the newly implanted lens in the proper position. Laser surgery is required to remove these opacifications and restore clear vision.

Why Do So Many People Develop Cataracts?

In most body tissues, new, healthy cells are constantly replacing worn-out cells. The lens of the eye, however, experiences no turnover of cells at all-which means that the ones you have when you are born are the ones that you have to last you your lifetime. This is why we need to keep our cells, tissues and blood system nourished with whole food supplements, eye supplements and whole natural foods, and avoid the fast food, sugar, white flour, junk food, high animal food intake of the western culture.

The lens of the eye is composed mostly of protein and water, which forms a structurally clear tissue allowing light to pass through and focus on the retina. As our health deteriorates, which causes rapid aging, the lens continues to grow and become less transparent to light. Long term photo (light) stress, oxidative stress, glycation and other factors can lead to severe distortions in the lens fiber proteins. The result is that proteins in the eye lens clump (crosslink), become oversaturated with water (water influx), and rupture in the cell fiber wall (bleb formation). All of this structural damage to lens proteins eventually creates opacity (inhibiting light transmission), which by definition is a cataract. Glycation or diabetes (sugar in the blood) is mainly causes by eating high glycemic foods, such as, sugar, white flour and fast foods and processed and packaged foods. High animals foods also put stress on the pancreas, causing inflammation, which stops the pancreas from secreting insulin; the result—diabetes, cataracts, glaucoma and macular eye degeneration. Inflammation, along with a high intake of liquids, coffee, pop, juices, common chemicalized tap water, all contribute to what Chinese Medicine calls Damp Heat. Heat is inflammation, and the dampness comes from drinking far too many liquids before, during and after meals, and in between. Excess water in the system weakens the kidneys and bladder, and expands the colon (large intestines) causing bloat. And this excess water and liquid intake travels up to the brain and eyes, where it water-logs or saturates the brain (brain edema), or water on the brain, and finally effects the vision (watery eyes, pressure on the eyes (glaucoma), cataracts and macular degeneration. It all goes back to the foundation of eating whole food nutrition, and taking whole food supplements to preserve and protect our eyes, organs and health. **(See Appendix I: 20 Secret Keys to Health and Longevity).**

If one does not know how to eat, what to eat, when to eat and other constructive life health habits, there will be no hope of maintaining healthy clear vision and super health for very long. Earlier chapters in this book go into detailed explanations on following daily health habits, body typing, supplements, exercise and positive mental attitude. Re-read those chapters again to get a thorough understanding of how your intricate biological system operates. Then you will avoid most of the pitfalls of being human, and take charge of your health and well-being.

What Causes Cataracts

Eye doctors say ultraviolet (UV) radiation is a risk factor for cataract formation. That may be true to a point. But, I don't totally agree with this evaluation. Excessive UV exposure may increase free radical formation in the lens, only if the person is consuming and saturating their bodies with lots of high sugar foods, white flour, lots of animal meat, animal fats, rancid fats and processed foods. How do we know this for sure. Look at the South Sea Islanders and people living out in nature, running around barefoot all day long in the sun, with few clothes on—none of these natural people get cataracts, unless they start eating a modern western diet. That won't happen if they stay in their natural environment and eat mostly foods from the land, mainly organic foods—fruits and vegetables, whole grains, seeds, nuts and beans, with only a minimum of animal foods. Once foods are refined, over time, health begins to decline rapidly, and so does eye health and vision. The body and eyes can overcome the damaging free radicals with antioxidant foods in the diet, plus super eye supplements as written in this book.

Scientists and clinical studies have proven that poor nutrition and cataract formation go hand in hand. People who increase specific target nutrients, lower their risk of cataracts, glaucoma and macula problems. Diabetics are directly effects by high blood sugar and oxidative free-radical stress. This is called glycation. This is all causes by a highly refined diet and lack of exercise.

Glycation is the binding of sugars to proteins, which causes the resulting glycated proteins to produce 50 times more free radicals than non-glycated proteins. This heightened oxidative stress works, in turn, to accelerate glycation reactions-a vicious cycle. The end result of uncontrolled glycation is rapid organ aging and increased risk of a number of age-related diseases. Glycated proteins trigger a process called cross-linking, where proteins become bound together, causing them to become inflexible and less able to function in physiological systems. This high oxidative stress comes from eating a diet high in animal proteins, including meat, chicken, turkey, fish, eggs, cheese, butter, milk and other dairy foods, sugar and junk food—high glycemic foods. Excess protein in the body turns into toxic residue, as endol, skatol, uric acid crystals, putrefaction, and this burdens the entire body with disease causing by-products of metabolism. This internal toxic soup scenario reaches the blood, brain and eyes, causing degeneration of the body and aging of the eyes.

Glycation plays a role in non-diabetics, especially high in sugars and refined carbohydrates eaters, or people with higher than normal blood sugar levels, but not high enough to be diabetic. Diabetes also can increase an enzyme (aldose reductase), probably from c-reactive protein and sugar in the diet, which clouds up the eye lens.

Taking bioflavonoids, and especially Quercetin, has been shown to reduce cataracts. Green vegetables and green food supplements, such as, green barley, spirulina, blue green algae, wheat grass, alfalfa, chlorella etc., can go a long way to nourish and prevent many health and eye problems.

Nuclear Cataract Formation

Nuclear Cataract Formation, is mainly caused by oxidative stress, of which a big cause is free radicals from rancid oils, excessive consumption of sugar products, trans fats, junk fast food oils, chemical sweeteners such as, aspartame (nutra sweet etc., and the latest one sucralose (chemically extracted form of white sugar0, which is damaging to health, and proper brain and eye function. Nuclear cataracts are caused by the same cause over years of poor eating habits and the above toxic food substances that damage the eye lens. Free radical oxidation in the eyes and brain is controlled and slowed down by a healthy diet, food, herbs and supplements that reduce oxidative stress, which reduce and neutralize free radical damage.

Reducing these free radical agents requires energy from healthy eating and living, outdoor walking, exercise, and eye exercises to circulate the blood to the brain and eyes, cells and tissues of the body. Healthy living and eating builds up fiber cells in the eye lens that lack mitochondria. The central eye lens fiber cells are delicately balanced, and can easily be weakened and damaged by an excess intake of high animal fats and proteins, sugar products of all kinds, and an excess amount of close work, like reading and computer work for hours on end. We are now seeing more eye problems, including cataracts and macula degeneration than ever before, especially in people who are tied to inside computers, television screens or video games, and also reading for hours at a time. This causes loss and lack of oxygen to the brain and eyes, along with poor food choices, stress, coffee, alcohol and tobacco—all causes of poor health, poor vision, and eye diseases.

The eyes take all the abuse that the mind and body give it, as they are delicate windows through which the brains sees and the soul looks out into the world. Excessive animal proteins accumulate in the eye lens and reduce enzyme activity, oxygen and blood circulation, causing cataracts and blurry vision. The eye lens is made to last over a hundred years, but cataracts are seen now by 40 or 50 years of age.

Cortical Cataract Formation

Unlike nuclear cataracts, cortical cataracts show disorganization of fiber cell structure. This is mainly caused by loss of calcium balance, protein accumulation and lack of antioxidant protection from glutathione in the body. Loss of calcium balance is caused by an excessive intake of animal proteins, including dairy products, which reduce calcium from being absorbed in the body. The more animal protein one eats, the less calcium the body absorbs. Protein reduces calcium in the blood and body and eyes. Most people are intolerant to the lactose in dairy products, so all the dairy that is consumed crystallizes and hardens as mucous in the eyes, joints, bones, causing cataracts, eye diseases, arthritis and bone degeneration.

Dairy products are not food for humans, only for the baby calf, which has to grow to a few hundred pounds in a year or two. Cow's milk is perfect for the calf, as it needs the high calcium and phosphorus that milk contains. But, when humans consume dairy products, poor health, i.e., eye disease, mucous in the eyes, coughing up mucous, colds, flu, asthma, bronchitis and pneumonia are the disastrous result. Cut out the dairy products and watch your vision and health zoom! No one can prove it to you, except you. Dairy and other animal products can easily cause oxidative damage to the eyes and lens. If you eat animal foods, keep them to no more than 10% of your total diet.

How to Protect the Eye Lens and Overcome Cataracts

We know much now about how cataracts are caused, and what nutrients are needed to stop the onslaught of this dreaded eye condition, which can lead to blindness. Prevention has been shown to prevent cataracts, and avoid surgery. Preventative target nutrition can also help glaucoma and aging macular malfunction.. Effective Nutrients at protecting against cataract, glaucoma and macular problems, **include carnosine, glutathione, taurine and cysteine; the antioxidant vitamins C, A and E; and vitamin B2 (riboflavin).** Here is how each of these nutrients helps protect the eyes against loss of vision.

Carnosine: Positive Eye and Health Free-Radical Scavenger Supplement
Carnosine inhibits formation of advanced glycation end products (AGEs) and protects normal proteins from the toxic effects of existing AGEs. Eye drops containing N-acetyl-L-carnosine can delay vision senescence in humans: effective in 100% of primary senile cataract cases and 80% of mature senile cataract cases. N-acetyl-L-carnosine enter the aqueous and lipid parts of the eye and prevent and repair light-induced breaks to DNA strands. N-acetyl-L-carnosine eye drops are approved for human use in Russia for the treatment of many eye diseases. **Brite Eyes II** is an advanced eye formula that contains 1% N-acetyl-L-carnosine in a soothing eye drop. A suggested oral dose of carnosine is 500-1000 mg daily. (Sachs) Carnosine is a free radical scavenger in the eyes. Carnosine helps maintain membrane function, fatty acids and cellular structure in the lens and eye. It prevents advanced glycation or protein cross-links. Carnosine stops glycation in its tracks, binding up protein on sugar molecules that causes the glycation process. This is the number one supplement acknowledged worldwide by nutritional researchers. Carnosine stops the toxic protein breakdown in the brain of Alzheimer's patients. It creates balance and homeostasis in the brain by neutralizing copper-zinc in the brain. It can prevent or reverse cataracts.

The topical form of N-acetyl-L-carnosine (time-released carnosine), which prevents DNA damage from poor nutrition and UV radiation, which repairs the DNA. Chinese and Russian studies found carnosine to be 80% to 100% effective, in beginning and long standing cataracts, respectively. They used a one percent solution of N-acetyl-carnosine, two times a day.

The research shows that N-acetyl-carnosine is a highly important super nutrient supplement to prevent cataracts. It is also an anti-aging nutrient that functions in many areas of the body to protect and prevent internal organ systems damage.

Glutathione, Vitamin E, NAC and Alpha Lipoic Acid Protect the Eyes from Damage. Oxygen in the eye lens is lower in diseased eyes, due to free radicals oxidative damage from ATP metabolism. Glutathione in the body protects this oxidative damage from happening. Glutathione is a special protein (a tripeptide) consisting of three amino acids: glutamic acid, cysteine, and glycine. Glutathione concentration is high in the lens, and it reduces oxidative damage. As glutathione is reduced in the lens, cataracts are formed and get worse over time.

Glutathione acts as a free radical scavenger in the eye lens, to help reduce cataracts. Glutathione goes directly to the center of the lens where it is needed, while the oxidized (used up) glutathione concentrates in the lens surface, causing the cloudy lens or cataract formation. As a result, older lens' have more free radical oxidative stress, which cause vision problems and eye diseases of all kinds.

Glutathione can benefit lens function by:

☯ Preserving the physicochemical integrity of proteins in the lens
☯ Maintaining action of the sodium-potassium transport pump and molecular integrity of lens fibers (protein)
☯ Maintaining molecular integrity of lens fiber membranes and acting as a free radical scavenger to protect membranes and enzymes from oxidation
☯ Preventing free-radical-induced photochemical generation of harmful by-products
☯ Glutathiione is high in healthy eyes and low in cataract eyes. Glutathione maintains the water balance in the lens. It is synthesized in the lens (and elsewhere) and is essential to normal metabolism.

A suggested glutathione dose is 500 mg daily. (Sachs)
Reactivating oxidized vitamin C, improves antioxidant capability in the lens. (Sachs)

Glutathione is found mainly in the eye lens. It protects the proteins and enzymes important for lens flexibility and clarity against free radical damage.. Aging or damaged eye lenses from a lifetime of poor nutrition, which causes oxidative stress, lose glutathione. A weak glutathione pool is known to lead directly to reactions that cause cross-linking of proteins and lens clouding. **L-carnosine** and **vitamin E** are the super nutrients that researchers have found to protect and restore higher levels of glutathione. Super supplements of **NAC (n-acetyl-cysteine)** and **alpha lipoic acid** increase tissue levels of glutathione in the eye.

Taurine: Maintains Optimal Function and Structure of the Eyes
Researchers at the University of Maryland found that high levels of **taurine** are required in the eye to maintain optimal function and structure. It is shown to protect the lens against free radical damage.

Vitamin C: Protects against UV Radiation and Protects the Eye Fluids
Vitamin C Ascorbates, a more natural and absorbable form of Vitamin C, or high

Vitamin C foods, like rose hips, camo camo, acerola,, Amla (Ayurvedic healing fruit), and many other fruits and vegetables, protect the lens from oxidative damage. Vitamin C is 30 to 50 higher in the eye lens than in the blood. Natural Vitamin C reacts quickly and efficiently with free radicals and other oxidants in the aqueous humor and lens, preventing damage to lens proteins, lipids, and nucleic acids. (Robert Sachs)

Vitamin C is found in high concentrations in eyes of animals active during day light hours; low concentrations are found in nocturnal animals. Prior to cataract formation, vitamin C concentrations significantly drop. Vitamin C provides protective benefits for the lens by:

☙ Protecting the lens from photochemical oxidation
☙ Helping increase levels of glutathione
☙ Supporting delicate membranes regulating transport of nutrients and ions (minerals and electrolytes) into the lens
☙ Protecting against damaging UV radiation and visible light
☙Protecting against superoxide radical, O_2- (known to be extremely destructive in every cell). (Sachs).
A suggested dose of vitamin C is 500 mg daily. (Sachs)

Vitamin C helps reduce cataract formation, and protects against UV radiation. Adequate Vitamin C from fruits and vegetables, plus 1,000 to 2,000 mg. of Vitamin C Ascorbates with Bioflavonoids reduces or prevents cataract development. The longer you use Vitamin C the more protection you receive. Vitamin C is found in high levels in the aqueous humor (the fluid that fills the eyeball and filters light as it passes through to the retina) and the corneal epithelium (the outer layer of the front of the eyeball). More benefits of clear vision come also from eating a whole foods diet, avoiding sugars, refined carbs and high fat animal foods, along with a moderate amount of natural Vitamin C Ascorbates. You will need less Vitamin C supplementation if your diet is not high in refined foods. The higher your diet is in high natural whole foods and minerals, the less you will need to rely on excessive use of Vitamin C. When the body is stressed and inflamed with refined foods, sugar and meat, you will, more than likely, need more Vitamin C to counteract the toxic by-products from those foods. It is always better to follow nature's plan, then suffer with the toxic plan of man.

Riboflavin: Buffers Free Radicals in the Eyes
Vitamin B2 (riboflavin) aids glutathione in the eye lens, and reduces free radical damage, which reduces or neutralizes peroxide free radicals in the eyes. Deficiency of glutathione weakens the antioxidant defense system in the lens.

Consuming tons of junk food, toxic oils, animal fats, combined with excessive exposure to ultraviolet (UV) light, destroys riboflavin. B-vitamins must be replaced daily. Riboflavin deficiency is a prime cause of photosensitivity making the eye more sensitive to UV damage. Use 50 to 150 mg of riboflavin daily to help reduce light sensitivity.
Vitamin B2, (riboflavin) removes oxidized glutathione, (used up) glutathione, a by-product in the process of buffering free radicals and has become a free radical-bearing

molecule itself, from the lens of the eye. Ophthalmology Research in the March 2000 issue of the journal Ophthalmology found the B-vitamins to protect against cataracts. Riboflavin, along with other B-complex vitamins provides a considerable degree of protection against cataracts, glaucoma and macular degeneration. When buying B-vitamins, purchase 100% whole food B-complex, which are grown on food based enzymes. They are not synthetic, therefore lower in total milligrams than the high milligram high dosed B-complex vitamins that are made from a chemical process of coal tar. High dosed B-complex may stimulate you to feel good for awhile, but they are far from natural, and you get diminishing returns after a month or two. The body cannot recognize a coal tar chemical product internally, so it tries to "kick it out," therefore you get dark yellow urine, and you may get withdrawal symptoms if you stop using them, or cut them off quickly. It is better to use whole food B-complex supplements from companies such as, Mega Foods, Systemic Formulas, or New Chapter. They nourish your entire body, without leaving toxic residues in your lungs, kidneys, colon and liver. The liver has to filter out all the synthetic, chemicalized and toxic substances coming in from the diet and environment. It is best not to put more chemicals into your body if you can help it. Use the supplements from these three great companies, and you'll be safe and healthy.

Vitamin E and Selenium: Restores Glutathione Levels
Selenium works with alpha-lipoic acid to increase cellular concentrations of glutathione, which protects the eye lens from free radical damage. Taking 400–800 IU daily of vitamin E and 200–400 mcg daily of selenium is prudent to protect the lens from cataract formation and maintain overall good health. (Sachs)

High levels of vitamins protect the eyes, while low levels are found in cataracts. An Italian University study discovered that high levels of vitamin E restored glutathione levels in degenerated rat eye lenses. German researches found that low vitamin E levels in the body and eyes, along with UV radiation exposure caused increased eye damage. Eating whole foods, with super foods such as, wheat germ, whole rice bran, nutritional imported yeast, whole grains, and taking a natural source of Vitamin E made from wheat germ oil or rice bran oil will restore your Vitamin E levels in your eyes and body. Stay away from the cheap Vitamin E made from soy oil. Read labels, and purchase a high quality Vitamin supplements from Carlson Company or Unique E Inc. Carlson has one or two Vitamin E supplements made only from wheat germ, and Unique Company is made with wheat germ oil exclusively. Carlson also has a couple Vitamin E's made from soy oil–avoid those at all costs–even though they are cheaper. You get what you pay for. Buyer beware, especially in health food stores. Not everything is natural or wholesome there, so you can fall asleep in a somnambulistic trance in a health store, thinking everything in there is good for you. Not so! Read labels and know what you are buying at all times. New Chapter has a good Vitamin E.

Alpha-Lipoic Acid
Alpha-lipoic acid can help prevent cataract formation from lack of glutathione synthesis. Alpha-lipoic acid has been shown to reduce cataract formation by 40%, and also to protect the lens from vitamins C, E, and glutathione lose in the eye. Without these

supplements, the eyes cannot uptake these supplements. 150-300 mg per day of lipoic acid is suggested. 500 mg of Vitamin C, along with plenty of steamed and raw vegetables and fruits and soaked seeds, nuts and grains. Also, 200 to 400 units of high quality Vitamin E from Rice Bran oil or Wheat Germ Oil.

N-Acetyl-Cysteine and Garlic
A combination of daily disulfide (a major organosulfide in garlic oil) and N-acetyl-cysteine (NAC) completely prevented cataract development in animals. NAC assists in glutathione production because it is a source of cysteine, one of the three amino acids in this tripeptide. A suggested dose of NAC is 600 mg daily. Take two enteric coated garlic caplets daily. I like Garlicin or Allermax garlic supplements. Make sure they are "enteric coated" so they by pass the stomach acids, which reduces their effectiveness.

Melatonin
Melatonin is an antioxidant that help stop cataract development. Animals studies showed melatonin inhibited cataract formation, due to free-radical scavenging or through stimulation of glutathione production. Melatonin production slows after age 40, but by age 60 virtually no melatonin is produced at a time when most cataracts develop. A suggested dose of melatonin is 500 mcg to 3 mg at bedtime. (Sachs).

Lens Protein Protection

Vitamin B6
Vitamin B6 (pyridoxine) is needed for amino acid and protein metabolism, absorbing vitamin B12, and proper synthesis of nucleic acids. Its coenzyme is required for many reactions of amino acids and related metabolic functions. Vitamin B6 is suggested for nutritional support for cataract patients. A suggested dose of vitamin B6 is 50-250 mg daily.(Sachs). Get the whole food B6 from New Chapter or Mega Food.

Acetyl-L-Carnitine
Acetyl-L-carnitine: an amino acid that strengthens cellular metabolism of fatty acids. During aging, mitochondria (energy-producing organelles within the cell) begin to deteriorate, resulting in accumulation of cellular debris and eventual cell death. Acetyl-L-carnitine can diminish advanced glycation end product (AGE) damage that leads to cataract formation. Acetyl-L-carnitine can acetylate (deactivate) potential glycation sites on crystallins and protect them from glycation-mediated protein damage. A suggested dose of acetyl-L-carnitine arginate is 3-4 capsules daily. (Sachs)

Aminoguanidine
Aminoguanidine inhibits advanced glycation end products (AGEs) and may treat diabetic cataracts. This product cannot protect the eyes by itself; blood sugar levels must be regulated by a good diet, exercise and a healthy lifestyle program, so that antiglycating agents such as aminoguanidine can protect against cataract. A suggested dose of aminoguanidine is 300 mg daily. Take this under a physician's supervision. It can inhibit vitamin B6 uptake so take B6 with it. **Note:** The Alteon Corporation (USA) has aminoguanidine (Pimagidine®) in stage III trials for diabetes.

Lens Metabolism Support

Bioflavonoids

Bioflavonoids are powerful inhibitors of the enzyme aldose reductase. If aldose reductase activity falls, sorbitol is not synthesized. This reduces the accumulation of water in the lens. The bioflavonoids quercetin, myrcetin, and kaempferol (from limes) specifically inhibit diabetic cataracts. Gingko is a widely used flavonoid that helps microcirculation to the eye and inhibits free radical damage, which cause cataracts. A suggested dose of gingko biloba is 120 mg daily. Take one or two capsules of bioflavonoids daily.

Inositol

Inositol nicotinate is a B-vitamin found in the lens. Inositol is an antioxidant that quenches the reactive oxygen and scavenging of glucose. Take Inositol with B-complex vitamins. A suggested dose of inositol is 250 mg daily.

Ocular Environment Support

Carotenoids, Vitamin A, Astaxanthin, Lutein, Zeaxanthin: Protects the Eye Retina

Astaxanthin, from ocean microalgae boosts immunity and energy to the entire body, and is 20 times more potent than the other carotenoids. It protects the the liver and helps to improve vision, **(See Appendix H).** Vitamin A or beta carotene from carrots protects the eye retina. Vitamin A protects against cataract formation. Vitamin C, E, and A regenerates oxidized glutathione. Antioxidants work synergistically, boosting each other, as they also are oxidized in the process of buffering free radicals. Vitamin A is also used topically for contact lens problems and topical eye problems. Carotenoids are fat-soluble, yellowish pigments found in some plants, algae, carrots and, red peppers and photosynthetic bacteria. Carotenoids are light-gathering pigments that provide protection from the toxic effects of oxygen-free radicals and singlet oxygen which are generated in the presence of light and oxygen. Lutein and zeaxanthin are carotenoids found in high concentrations in the macula of the retina. Lutein and zeaxanthin protect the eye from age-related macular degeneration and cataract formation. Lutein is derived from dark green leafy vegetables (spinach, broccoli, kale, and collard greens). Zeaxanthin is found in yellow fruits and vegetables (corn, peaches, and mangoes). Suggested doses are 5 mg of zeaxanthin, 4 mg of astaxanthin, and 20 mg of lutein.

Coenzyme Q10

Coenzyme Q10 (CoQ10) is an antioxidant that protects the eyes from free-radical damage. A combination of antioxidants including CoQ10, Acetyl-L-carnitine, polyunsaturated fatty acids (PUFAs), and vitamin E improved macular degeneration in retinal pigment. Entire body glycation (excess sugar, white flour, animal fats, lack of exercise and shallow breathing) is a dysfunction that occurs throughout the body and produces damaging reactive free radical oxygen damage that cause eye disease, aging, and illness. Take 100-200 mg daily of CoQ10 daily, more if you have heart problems.

Potassium and Magnesium

A lens with cataracts has low concentrations of potassium and magnesium. Potassium and magnesium are often reduced in diseased and aging humans. Take 400 mg of potassium and 800 mg of magnesium citrate, which will increase the availability of these minerals to the lens and protect your arteries. Also, consuming plenty of fresh fruits and vegetables increases potassium and magnesium levels in the eyes, blood and body.

Gingko and Bilberry
Gingko biloba extract is an antioxidant, increases circulation to the optic nerve and has exhibited potential anti-cataract ability. Bilberry (from Vaccinium myrtillus fructus) is a proanthocyanidin, historically used for eye conditions, including glaucoma, cataracts, macular degeneration, diabetic retinopathy, and retinitis pigmentosa. Gingko biloba and bilberry may restore micro-capillary circulation. Suggested doses are Gingko biloba, 120 mg daily, and bilberry 100 mg daily. After taking Ginkgo and bilberry for a month; taking 400 mcg of selenium, 500 mg of glutathione, and 300 mg of alpha-lipoic acid daily has been suggested

SUPPLEMENTAL MEDICINE
Overview of Cataracts

When cataracts formation impairs your vision, they can be removed by surgery and a lens implant is put in its place. For most people, cataract surgery is effective and successful. Nutritional therapy is the best preventative of cataracts. There are no drugs to treat cataracts. Find out what is causing your cataracts: oxidative stress, free radical production, the breakdown and aggregation of lens proteins, dysfunction of metabolism in the lens, and inability to maintain a healthy ocular environment. Natural supplemental nutritional therapy is helpful for all these conditions. Also, as suggested in the beginning of this Chapter, proper eating habits, fasting, eating organic foods whenever possible, getting outdoor exercise, breathing exercises, yoga, reducing stress and staying away from refined sugar, white flour products, excessive consumption of animal foods and cutting way back on dairy products, or cutting them out altogether, will go a long way to reducing and preventing cataract formation from occurring in the first place.

Free Radical Reduction
Metabolic Changes and Cataract

Aging eyes undergo metabolic changes that predispose it to cataracts. This is from lack of oxygen and nutrients, which make the eyes subject to free-radical damage. Protect your eyes by taking antioxidants: such as, glutathione and vitamin C. This helps increase antioxidants in the eye, which neutralizes free radicals. Cataract formation comes on from the breakdown that regulates utilization of glutathione and vitamin C and/or decreases their concentration in the lens and surrounding structures. (Sachs).

Hydrogen Peroxide and Cataract

Cataract formation is initiated by the free-radical hydrogen peroxide found in the aqueous humor. Hydrogen peroxide oxidizes glutathione, or conversely, glutathione chemically reduces hydrogen peroxide, ultimately damaging the energy-producing system of the eye and allowing sodium to leak into the lens. Excess sodium attracts water to maintain osmolality, which initiates the edema phase of a cataract. Normal body heat in the lens catalyzes oxidation of the lens' proteins, which become opaque and insoluble (similar to the process by which egg protein changes from clear to opaque upon cooking). Free radicals break down fatty acids in membranes and lens protein fibers, generating more free radicals. This cross-links (or denatures or breaks down) the laminate-like structural proteins inside the lens capsule. The lens capsule can swell or shrink (dehydrate) and these changes in pressure breaks lens fiber membranes, forming microscopic spaces that trap water and debris.

Metabolism Support: Key Components

Powerful eye supplements are glutathione and vitamin C. In particular glutathione is required to protect mature lens fiber cells from free radical damage. Vitamin C Ascorbates with bioflavonoids helps to protect the lens from oxidative damage. Avoid Vitamin C from ascorbic acid. This is a chemically extracted vitamin C from high fructose corn syrup.

Protection from Free Radicals: The Glutathione Mechanism

Nutritional supplements reduce the risks of developing cataracts and slow or reverse cataract growth. Eye blood circulation is slow, so you will have to get the oxygen and blood circulating to your eyes and head with lying on a slant board with head lower, breathing deeply through your nose and feel the oxygen seeping up into your eye cavity and brain. Massage around your eyes on the forehead and arch of the eye. Gently massage closed eyelids. Also, place a slice of cucumber over each eye, with a luke warm face cloth over that for 15 minutes daily. The most important nutrients that stimulate antioxidant activity of glutathione, include vitamins C, B2, E, selenium, alpha lipoic acid, melatonin, N-acetyl-cysteine (NAC) with garlic, and glutathione.

Lens Protein Protection and Cellular Metabolism Maintenance

Proteins deep in the lens are generated during embryogenesis and must retain functionality for many decades. Lack of protein stability leads to formation of a cataracts. Once the lens forms in the embryo, proteins are only synthesized in the outermost fiber cells close to the lens surface. Accumulated damage to the proteins, from excess sugars, fats, aspartame, splenda, sucraclose, white flour and animal fats and animals proteins, causes loss of enzyme activity and increases protein aggregation, a product of cataract formation. Damage to proteins is, I believe, due to excessive intake of animal proteins, all sugars and chemical sugar substitutes, poor digestion, lack of enzymes, overeating, lack of hydrochloric acid (HCL) in the stomach to break down protein foods, lack of exercise, stress, excess alcohol, tobacco and too many chemicalized and processed foods in the diet. This is the major cause of the glycation or sugar metabolism process of the body, which adversely affects the eyes and vision.

The Glycation Process

Glycation damages lens proteins and greatly causes diabetic cataract formation and retinopathy. Glycation occurs when proteins react with sugars and form advanced glycation end products (AGEs). Proteins strongly bind to sugars, compromising the function of that protein. AGEs are biochemically altered proteins, DNA, and lipids with damaged biochemical properties. (Sachs). Nutritional supplements that help decrease breakdown of lens proteins and help maintain cellular metabolism include vitamin B6, acetyl-L-carnitine (ALC), aminoguanidine, bioflavonoids, inositol, and carnosine.

Maintaining a Healthy Ocular Environment

Cataract formation and aging go together, closely tied to increased oxidative stress, with a reaction of free radical attacks, and inefficient metabolic processes. Oxidation and glycation happens faster in the eye lens than anywhere else in the body. The lens consists of multiple layers of cells without the usual cellular organelles for energy production and other regenerative mechanisms for cellular bio-stability. Lens fiber cells dependent upon a small number of lens surface cells and surrounding cells for support. Over time these support mechanisms require increased nourishment and more antioxidants. (Sachs).

Aging (declining health), causes inefficiency of these supporting eye mechanisms. However, through optimal nutritional and supplemental intake, it is possible to reduce and prevent oxidative damage, and maintain high levels of antioxidants and cellular eye metabolism to optimize lens health. Aging and oxidative stress affects the whole system. Free radicals can be reduced in the eye through proper diet and lifestyle, thereby increasing overall health and well being.

SUMMARY

This nutritional and supplement protocol can help you protect your vision and prevent or slow down cataract formation. This information on cataracts and nutritional supplements should enable the reader to understand the beneficial effects of nutrition on cataract prevention.

Scientific Summary

Conventional treatment is removal of the eye lens, and replace it with an artificial lens. On the other hand, many physicians, researchers, and nutritional scientists have a more positive view of cataract prevention and treatment. This holistic approach to maintain healthy lens function and eye health includes awareness of risk factors (e.g., smoking, alcohol, sugar, white flour, processed oils, compliance with a sensible diet (e.g., low-fat, high-fiber), exercising, and nutritional therapy specifically for the eye.

Preventing Cataracts, Glaucoma and
Macula Degeneration in the First Place

You have been shown that individual nutrients can reduce cataract risk, along with a whole foods natural diet, low in refined sugars, animal fats, animal proteins and refined carbs, plus an increase in consumption of high fiber foods such as, whole grains, fruits, vegetables, seeds, nuts, grains, sprouts. We need about 25 to 30 grams of fiber daily, and you won't get that much eating the Standard American Diet (SAD). I call it the

Standard American Disease Diet (SADD). Along with a whole food eating program, a good exercise and walking routine, and you'll see dramatic improvement.

You can improve your chances of reducing and preventing eye problems with a multiple approach of these super-supplements: Natural Vitamin C Ascorbates or whole food vitamin C from New Chapter or Mega Foods, taurine, alpha lipoic acid, cysteine and riboflavin. Use a topical application (eye drops) of carnosine, vitamin A and vitamin E directly into the eye. Carnosine, vitamin A and vitamin E are also important nutrients to consume internally. Eat plenty of green super-food powders, raw and steamed greens.

Symptoms of Cataracts Formation

The progression of Cataracts will show the following symptoms:
1. Color blindness or altered color vision. 2. Cloudy vision, like looking through astained glass window. 3. Sun sensitivity or bright lights from oncoming cars. 4. Increasingly blurred vision. 5. You require more light to see things clearly. 6. Cover one eye and you see double vision. 7. Hard to see in the dark. 8. One eye can see more light than the other eye.

Cataracts come quicker if you:
- Develop diabetes.
- Exposed to UV radiation and eat a nutrient poor, fiber-less, junk food diet.
- Use topical drugs, steroid drugs, marijuana, pharmaceutical drugs or street drugs
- Are a heavy smoker now or in the past, (This also includes Marijuana).
- Consume poor nutrition
- Do not exercise

Supplement Recommendations

Lutein: 20 mg, one daily
Astaxanthin, 4 mg, one daily
Glutathione: 500 mg, one daily
Vitamin C: 500 mg, one daily
Vitamin B2: Coenzymated B2 by "<u>Source Naturals</u>," 25mg, 2 daily
Selenium: (Yeast bound), 200–400 mcg, one daily Never use synthetic selenium
Vitamin E: 400 IU daily. Mixed Vitamin E Tocotrienols (d-alpha, d-beta, d-delta, d-gamma) is a good choice, one daily, or Gamma E Mixed Tocopherol w/Sesame Lignans, one daily. Take mixed Tototrienols one day and mixed Tocopherols the next.
R-dihydro-lipoic acid: 150–300 mg daily
N-acetyl-cysteine (NAC): 600 mg, one daily
Melatonin: 300 mcg–3 mg at bedtime
Vitamin B6: P-5-P Coenzyme B6 Complex by "<u>Now Foods</u>", 50 mg, two daily
Acetyl-L-carnitine arginate: three-four capsules daily
Aminoguanidine: 150–300 mg, one daily
Carnosine: 500–1000 mg daily
Brite Eyes II: One-two drops in each eye daily

Perfect Eyesight

Lutein Plus Powder: (Life Extension Foundation). One tablespoon daily taken with a fatty meal.
Super Zeaxanthin 4mg with Lutein 20mg: One-two capsules daily.
Coenzyme Q10: 100–200 mg daily
Potassium: 400 mg daily, but consult your physician
Magnesium: 800 mg daily
Gingko biloba: 120 mg daily
Bilberry: 100 mg daily
Kyolic Reserve Garlic: 1 to 3 capsules daily

Seven Steps to Powerful Heatlh

(Excerpted from Article Archives at www.youngagain.com). (Free books on pdf and articles by Roger Mason, Biochemist Researcher. With elucidation and commentary by Health Reseacher, aka R.T.Lewis (Robert Lewanski)
There are seven vital steps to take if you want excellent health and long life.
Do the best you can to follow all of them.

1. A whole food based diet—whole grains, legumes, vegetables, fruits, soaked seeds and nuts, and fish if you want. Meat must be kept to 5-10% of diet to keep your acid-alkaline balance. Diet is the core program to your health. Diet and exercise prevents disease; supplements and herbs are adjuncts to a healthy lifestyle. Diet is everything.

2. Proven double-blind, scientifically tested supplements are powerful when you're eating correctly for your specific body type, and following the natural laws of health as stated in this book. There are only about twenty scientifically proven supplements for those over forty, and eight for those under forty. Use the Systemic Healing Formulas, from systemicformulas.com, and the ones from www.youngagain.com.

3. Get your natural hormone balance checked, as an important step for maintaining youthful hormones. Your fourteen basic hormones are described in books for FREE pdf download at www.youngagain.com. You can get tested through saliva and hair samples through the mail, without a doctor. Get the Hormone TEST KIT from www.youngagain.com. You can save 100 to 200 dollars, with the Self-Test Kit ($55.00).

4. Exercise is next to a good diet, as stated in the 20 Keys to Health and Longevity. (See **APPENDIX I**) at back of this book. Walking, mini-trampoline, light weights etc.

5. Fasting is the most powerful healing method known to man. Just fast from dinner to dinner on water one day a week. Join Roger Mason's monthly Young Again two day fast. The fasting calendar is at www.youngagain.org. It is the last weekend of every month.

6. Avoid prescription drugs, except *temporary* antibiotics or pain medication during an emergency. The only exception is insulin for type 1 diabetics who have no operant pancreas. Drugs are worse than the illness, and cause terrible side-effects, which make you even more sick.

7. The last step is to limit or end any bad habits such as alcohol, coffee, recreational drugs, or sugared desserts. You don't have to be a saint, but you do have to be sincere.

With these seven steps you can prevent and cure "incurable" illnesses naturally like cancer, diabetes, heart disease and others without drugs, surgery, or radiation. This is done by eating whole natural foods, and enhancing your hormones with natural supplements to "youthful" levels, thereby turning back the aging process many years.

For More Information

Contact the National Eye Health Education Program of the National Institutes of Health, (301) 496-5248, or the American Society of Cataract Surgery, (703) 591-2220 .

Product Availability

Go to **www.momentum98.com** for some of the products listed. This is a wholistic health supplement and body care distributor website. Phil Wilson has Ayurvedic and Chinese Herbal tonics and powerful vitamin, mineral, enzyme, tonic supplements—some of the top products in the country. You can also call to place your order after viewing all the products: Call **Phil Wilson** or staff, **800-533-4372**, and tell them you read it here in Perfect Eyesight. Mention my name, and you'll get a special deal on the RELAX FAR INFRA RED ("CHI LIGHT HEALING") SUANA. Use the Sauna in combination with the Oxy/Oz Ozone Machine from momentum98.com, to boost your entire immune system, health, metabolism and eyesight with healing light energy, and pure oxygen—right down to your cellular DNA level. This will be your best investment to stay young and vital, and improve your vision. **(See Appendix F and J).**

For further discounted supplements and free books on diabetes, cholesterol, weight loss, health, prostate health and more, go to: **www.youngagain.com** or **www.youngagain.org**. You will learn a wealth of knowledge from this site. There is archived articles and free book downloads. And if you order any supplements from this site, you will receive a free book of your choice, 9 or 10 books listed there.

Also, go to www.systemicformulas.com, the most powerful synergistic and bio-energetic herbal formulas in the world that work like no other herbal supplements can. They are bio-balanced and resonate at high vibratory frequencies that match the frequencies of cells, tissues, organs, glands and bone. They can help clean up your cells, tissues, organs, right down to the DNA and Telomeres attached to the ends of your chromosomes. Systemic Formulas is that powerful!

Chapter Twelve

The Aging Eye and Macular Degeneration:
How You Can Protect Your Vision

Blindness is not inevitable, no matter how long you live. Aging eyes and macula degeneration don't just happen by themselves. Many factors come into play here. For instance, diet, exercise, outdoor activity, walking; how much close work you do; stress; sugar, sweets and chemical sweeteners; whole food supplements; eye supplements; eye herbs; liver herbs; is your blood circulation good; is your body flexible—all these play into how good your vision will be today, tomorrow or a hundred years from now. The eyes will age along with the body—if the body ages rapidly, the eyes will dim, weaken and lose their sight. . Degeneration of the body creates changes in eye health also. This often happens at mid-life. However, children are now developing weak and aged vision, due to all the close work, stress and fast food junk food. . By age 70, most people who suffer with ill health, also suffer from macular degeneration, glaucoma and/or cataract. Diabetic retinopathy, is also caused from overall poor health, which affects the body, the mind and the eyes, and is also a major cause of visual degeneration among adults, and children too. Many eye diseases can be prevented with lifestyle changes. A scientific body of wisdom indicates that many supplemental antioxidants and anti-glycating agents, like **carnosine**, help to prevent and treat eye disease. When poor health and weak vision set in, this causes reduced blood flow to the eye, thereby slowing down the assimilation and absorption of nutrients into the eye. This can be helped by topical treatments placed into the eye, (see previous chapter) to help protect against eye problems, such as cataracts and macula degeneration. This can help adults as well as children with eye problems.

Most people over 75 have cataracts, and most of them opt for cataract surgery. You can take action now to prevent eye diseases early in life, and enjoy good vision indefinitely, and never develop cataracts or other eye diseases.

Cataracts are a clouding of the lens of the eye, which reduces incoming light and results in vision deterioration. Reading and driving become difficult and sometimes impossible with this reduced light coming into the eyes. Eyeglasses need to be upgraded constantly in this condition. Twenty million people worldwide suffer from cataracts. More than 350,000 cataract operations are performed in the United States yearly.

Many people are born with minor lens opacities that never progress, while others progress to the point of blindness or surgery. Many factors influence vision and cataract development such as age, nutrition, medications and sunlight exposure. High blood pressure, kidney disease, diabetes or direct trauma to the eye can also cause cataracts.

The process of degenerating health due to poor diet and health habits, itself leads to certain metabolic changes that may predispose the lens to cataract development. Some of this occurs due to low supply of oxygen and nutrients, which leave the eye open to free radical damage. According to a 1983 report from the National Academy of Science, cataracts are initiated by free-radical hydrogen peroxide found in the aqueous humor. Free radicals such as hydrogen peroxide oxidize glutathione (GSH), destroy the energy-producing system of the eye, and allow leakage of sodium into the lens. Water follows the sodium, and the edema phase of the cataract begins. Then, body heat in the lens of the eye oxidizes (cooks) lens protein, and it becomes opaque and insoluble (similar to egg protein).

The good news is that cataract and macula degeneration can be slowed or prevented by the use of natural therapies and positive lifestyle changes, eating habits and powerful anti-oxidant supplements to change the internal environment of the body cells, blood and eye lens. Researchers at Brigham and Women's Hospital, Harvard Medical School, stated in the January/February 1999 issue of Journal of Association American Physicians that, "Basic research studies suggest that oxidative mechanisms may play an important role in the pathogenesis of cataract and age-related macular degeneration, the two most important causes of visual impairment in older adults." The researchers suggest preventing and preserving the eye lens with high antioxidant supplements to prevent eye degeneration and improve the overall health of the body.

Scientists report that supplements can reduce free-radical damage, which can return and reverse free radical damage. Although it is difficult to treat cataracts with oral antioxidants since there is only minimal blood circulation within the eye, compared to other parts of the body, nutritional supplements have been shown to reduce the risks of cataracts as well as slow or reverse their progression. However, oxygen and circulation can be brought to the eyes through yoga exercises, oxygen/ozone therapy, (see **Appendix J**), deep breathing, eye supplements and special eye drops, designed to bring oxygen to the eye lens. It has been scientifically shown that eye (cataract) degeneration can be slowed or stopped, and that oxygen filled blood can be brought to the eyes with the use of carotene and beta-carotene, astaxanthin, lycopene and lutein.

Age-Related Macular Degeneration (AMD)

The macula is the center of the retina. It takes in images from the environment and sends them via the optic nerve from the eye to the brain. The macula focuses central vision for seeing fine detail, reading, driving and recognizing facial features.

AMD is a condition in which the central portion of the retina (the macula) deteriorates. The cause is poor health, caused by unhealthy lifestyle, bad eating habits, stress and lack of exercise, smoking, alcohol etc. Macular degeneration affects more Americans than cataracts and glaucoma combined. There are two forms of macular degeneration: The dry eye and wet eye. This comes from either a dry internal body type system, such as a dry/hot Vata/Pitta body type (dry eye type), or a wet/damp Kapha body type (wet eye type), as discussed in previous chapters of this book. Both forms of dry or wet may affect both eyes simultaneously at different times, due to what foods are eaten, and certain body types. Usually central vision rather than peripheral vision is impaired. .

Conventional medical treatment programs cannot restore lost eyesight with either form of the disease. Leading researchers, however, are documenting the benefits of a more holistic approach in the treatment of AMD, Aging Macular Degeneration. Increase your physical fitness, improve nutrition (including a reduction in saturated fats), and abstain from smoking. Dietary supplementation of trace elements, antioxidants and vitamins is recommended for improving overall metabolic and vascular functioning. Early testing to find out your eye condition can move you in the correct wholistic vision care arena.(4)

Poor nutrition and decreased antioxidant supplementation is the major cause of eye degeneration. Lower glutathione levels in the blood and eye lens contributes to further eye problems. In addition, an increase of oxidized or damaged glutathione creates increased oxidation and aging vision. Glutathione protects retinal pigment from degenerating. Glutathione is concentrated in the lens, and has been shown to have a hydroxyl radical-scavenging function in lens epithelial cells.[5]

Diabetic Retinopathy

High blood sugar levels is associated with diabetes and blindness. Diabetic retinopathy is due to damage of the retinal blood vessels. This causes the ruptured vessels to leak fluid, restricting oxygen and blurring sight. As the disease progresses, the eye tries to form new vessels on the surface of the retina, which may also bleed or obscure sight by their presence. Controlling blood sugar is a good way to preventing or slow down the progression of diabetic retinopathy.

In glaucoma, (open-angle) the common form of the disease, drainage of the aqueous fluid is sluggish, so the backup causes the undue pressure in the eye. The pressure pinches the blood vessels that feed the optic nerve, causing the nerve to die over time.

In diabetics, the eye fluids change more rapidly than with just normal aging. These changes cause eye malfunction and retinal detachment. The vitreous body of the eye is composed of a fine network of hyaluronan gel, collagen, proteoglycans and fibronectin, all of which are susceptible to free radical damage brought on by high glycation, from eating a diet high in sugars and other high glycemic foods. Because of this nutritional and internal health insufficiency, and eye and organ weakness, the eyes cannot take sunlight and UV light, and weaken further.[6]

Toxic oxidation induced by glycation can wreak havoc on the eye. Protein glycation occurs when sugar molecules inappropriately bind to protein molecules, forming cross-links that distort the proteins and consequently render them useless. Glycation appears to increase oxidative processes, which may explain why both glycation and oxidation simultaneously increase with age. High blood sugar from high glycemic foods, ie, sugar, white flour, high fructose corn syrup, and chemical sweeteners, such as, aspartame, sucralose also increases glycation activity, which may also explain the various kinds of tissue damage that create advanced diabetes.

Glaucoma

Glaucoma results from the build-up of pressure in the aqueous humor, the liquid that fills the area between the cornea and the lens. Generally, the condition develops after age 40. A lack of antioxidants increase physical stress on the eye, and oxidation takes place.[7] Low antioxidant activity in lacrimal (tear) fluid and blood plasma coincides with glaucoma.[8] It also is noted that the rate of crystalline damage increases as antioxidants and protease activity declines with with poor body and eye health.[9] In glaucoma, drainage of the aqueous fluid is weak or slow, so it backs up causing eye pressure. This eye pressure pinches the blood vessels that feed the optic nerve, causing the nerve to die over time, and leading to decreased peripheral vision, tunnel *vision and* finally blindness. A rarer form of glaucoma is called narrow-angle or congestive glaucoma, whereby the flow of the aqueous liquid is blocked causing pressure to build up. This is all caused by poor nutrition, junk food, lack of exercise and blood circulation to the eyes and head. Super-nutrition eye supplements can go a long way to help reverse these conditions, along with a good healthy lifestyle program.

Focus on Improving Eye Health and Healthy Eating

Most eye doctors don't know what causes aging eye diseases. However, most eye diseases are caused by oxidative damage. The eye lens acts as a light filter for the retina. When poor nutrition (high sugar, white flour, high levels of polyunsaturated fatty acids, trans fats, like margarine, and other hardened vegetable oils, dairy foods and high glycemic foods) is constantly eaten, the eyes, brain and blood is put under chronic photo-oxidative stress. Because reactive oxidation takes place in the cellular metabolism of the eye, we see the eye weakening, clouding up, and degenerating into cataracts and glaucoma.[10]

Aging eyes are the result of cellular enzyme breakdown. Enzymes metabolize and detoxify hydrogen peroxide and other free radicals found in eye fluids.[11] Free radicals take over the aqueous fluid and bathe the lens of the eye, destroying enzymes that produce energy and maintain cellular metabolism. Free radicals also break down fatty molecules in membranes and lens fibers, generating more free radicals and creating a cross-linking (denaturing or breakdown) of the laminated-like structural proteins inside the lens capsule. The lens capsule has the ability to swell or dehydrate. In doing so, the increase and/or decrease in pressure can cause breaks in the lens fiber membranes, resulting in microscopic spaces in the eye in which water and debris can reside. This is all caused by high consumption of the SAD diet (Standard American Diet) of fast food, processed, denatured, packaged, frozen, chemicalized and sterilized, so-called "food." This junk food is not fit to feed animals, let alone humans.

Blood flow in the eye decreases with age because of poor lifestyle and eating habits, depriving them of crucial nutrients for proper function and antioxidant activity.[12] Vascular changes come about from poor health, which causes glaucoma, or so-called age-related macular degeneration. Researchers showed that retinal and central retinal artery blood flow significantly decreases as a person's health declines, along with age.{14} Health declines first, then aging eyes and physical aging follow in their shadow.

Preventing Degenerative Eye Disease
Scientific studies on eye aging has demonstrated that antioxidants such as Vitamin C Ascorbates, carotenoids and tocopherol, may protect against cataract formation.[1] A 5 year study of 3000 people from Wisconsin, aged 43 to 86 years old showed cataracts were 60% lower for those taking vitamins containing Vitamin C or E, over a 10 year span, as compared to those who didn't take these supplements.

A Harvard study showed a 19% lower cataract risk factor with those taking lutein and zeaxanthin.(16) These two eye carotenoid supplements are found in the macula, and they reduce free-radical formation from light and oxygen. The macula is the center of the retina, and gives the eye sharp detail. Macular pigment protects the retina by scavenging free radicals and also filtering out blue light, which can contribute to photochemical damage in weak eyes from poor nutrition and lack of outdoor exercise, and excessive stress and close work. Macular degenerated eyes always show lower levels of carotenoids in them.

A Russian study revealed that 64 patients who combined a program of hyperbaric oxygen and antioxidant supplements, over a five year span, improved eye function in 80% of the group. This is why the OxyOz Oxygen machine can help in getting pure oxygen into your organs, cells and eyes. (See **Appendix J**) for more information on this powerful OxyOz Ozone Oxygen machine, from www.momentum98.com.

A Baltimore Study discovered that tocopherol, carotene and ascorbates protect the eyes; especially alpha-tocopherol, which stopped eye degeneration in a France study.

Another free-radical scavenger and anti-glycating agent is (NAC) N-Acetyl-Carnosine. Out of 49 people, 60 or over, with cataracts, about 42% treated with a 1% solution of NAC drops, twice a day improved their eye lens clarity, 90 improved their visual acuity, and 89% were less glare sensitive.

The eye supplements that helps the macula pigment is lutein and zeaxanthin. Vitamin C is concentrated in the aqueous humor and corneal epithelium. Glutathione is strongly concentrated in the eye lens. Zinc is found in high concentrations in the retinal pigment epithelium (tissue behind the retina that nourishes the rods and cones, that allow the eyes to see images. These are all anti-glycating agents to help the eyes see clearly for a long time. This is also confirmed by the USDA, a Human Nutrition Research Center on Aging.

Of all the fruit and vegetables, corn contains the highest lutein, and orange sweet peppers have the highest zeaxanthin content, 37%. Organic, non-GMO corn contain the highest lutein and zeaxanthin, 85%. Egg yolk also has 85% carotenoid content, but eating too many eggs can cause a fatty liver and blocked arteries. So be careful of this one. Other foods with high carotenoid content are spinach, oranges, grapes, kiwi, zucchini and winter squashes 30% to 50%. Leafy green vegetables has 15% to 47% lutein, but a low 0 to 3% zeaxanthin content. So, eat plenty of dark green vegetables, steamed and raw.

The problem with taking oral eye supplements is getting their nutrient factors into the eye tissues where they are needed. Tests were shown that the nutrients got into the blood, but not into the eye lens. So this is where we need to get the blood circulation and oxygen into the eyes through vigorous outdoor walking, aerobics and light weight exercising. Use the Ozy/Oz Ozone Machine and Far InfraRed Sauna to get more oxygen into your eyes and brain. **Oxygen-Breathing-Eye Technique:** Lie on a slant-board, with head down, and do deep slow in-and-out breathing through the nose, and feel the breath go up into the brain and eye cavity. Yoga postures can also help in getting oxygen to the brain and eyes, i.e., the plough position and head stand. The plough position is when you lie on your back, and bring your legs up above your head, and hold your lower back with your palms as a brace to hold your spine in a vertical position; then do the deep belly breathing. Oxygen and blood flows to through the neck into the brain and eyes and face. Try it, and see what results you get. It won't hurt. Just be sure your blood pressure is normal before getting into any inverted body positions. If you can't do a "head stand," just bend over from the waist—breathe in-out. Another study done by the National Eye Institute showed 19% less vision loss by taking Vitamin C, E, beta carotene and zinc. The talk in the scientific arena is in giving topical treatment of antioxidants, which is a targeted delivery system of essential nutrients directly to the eyes. Time will tell on this question. Keep your mind open to new and improve eye health supplements and delivery systems.

Reversing Diabetes and Diabetic Related Eye Diseases Through Diet and Healthy Life-Style Habits

In actual real time dietary therapy, **Dr. Gabriel Cousens, MD**, at his healing resort in Arizona, has taken diabetic clients off of insulin in 4 days, and brought down his patient's blood sugar down to below 80, from over 150 to 200 points within four weeks. How is that for "real time" results. Go to **http://www.treeoflife.nu/**, which is the website to **The Tree of Live Rejuvenation Center in Patagonia, Arizona.** Anything that reduces high blood sugar levels and diabetes, will have a positive effect on vision also. Diet and health of the body directly impact one's vision and eye health. They go hand and hand. You can't have one without the other. If your diet is SAD (Standard American Diet) junk food and dead food, don't expect good health and clear vision. Just won't happen.

What Dr. Cousens recommends to lose weight, lose your diabetes, and get back your health and well being is a basic foundation vegan diet. Organic foods, high in minerals. Low glycemic index foods, and low insulin index foods, like plenty of vegetables, sprouts, quality proteins, lots of exercise, walking, yoga, and meditation. High glycemic and high insulin index foods are fast foods, white flour, white sugar, cakes, pies, candy, soft drinks, white bread, white noodles—most packaged and processed and non-organic foods—all fall into this disease producing category. Low glycemic/low insulin index foods actually reduce and reverse diabetes, and also help the vision to improve tremendously. What causes most disease in this "Culture of Death," as Cousens says, is high sweet sugary foods, high trans fatty foods and junk oils, high meat and dairy and animal fat intake, empty calorie foods, and high intake of pharmaceutical drugs. All of these "foods" and drugs cause physical degeneration of the body, eyes, mind and spirit.

What is a Low Insulin Index: How much a food raises insulin secretion in the pancreas. One-quarter pound of beef raises the insulin index equal to a quarter pound of sugar—it stresses and exhausts the pancreas and causes inflammation, which damages these sugar regulating organs. Whole vegetables, whole grains, whole beans, sprouts do not raise the insulin levels, therefore they are Low Insulin Index foods. The solution: decrease inflammation with a low sugar, low refined white flour, low animal fats and foods, and increase fiber to 25 to 30 grams a day. Most people eat 5 or less grams of fiber daily, therefore, they stay sick and overweight. Increase your fiber and you can cure your own diabetes and weight problems, and also improve your visual health at the same time. Excessive consumption of fruit, especially sweet fruit, like bananas, melons, oranges etc, can easily cause a reactive sugar to protein syndrome in some people, especially with lack of exercise; exercise burns off sugar and helps your internal organs metabolize foods more efficiently. Sugar and meat are the primary cause of diabetes and diabetic retinopathy. If you exercise, breathe deeply and sweat, your body requires more potassium and magnesium from fruits and vegetables. Without some form of exercise, you won't enjoy good health and good vision.

High glucose blood sugar or glycation is the culprit. And sugar, refined white flour carbs, meat animal foods, dairy and junk fast foods is the trigger factor in most all sugar problems, diabetes, hypoglycemia, weight, eye and health problems. Cousens' quotes Dr. Cleave, who talks about the 20 year rule: "Twenty years after junk food and refined fast food is brought into the culture, disease begins to occur—diabetes, cancer, blood diseases, bone disease, eye diseases and on and on."

Powerful Supplements to Optimize Your Eye Health

Vitamin E (mixed tocotrienols), Acetyl-l-carnitine, Vitamin C as calcium ascorbates, bioflavonoids, quercetin, Carnosine, Ornithine alpha-ketoglytarate, Calcium pyruvate, B complex vitamins, Glutathione, Beta carotene, Astaxanthin, Zeaxanthin, Lutein, Selenium (yeast bound), Zinc polynicotate, and Manganese.

Chapter 12 References
1. Taylor A. EXS 1992;62:266-279.
2. Schalch W. EXS 1992;62:280-298.
3. Winkler BS, et al. Mol Vis 1999 Nov 3;5:32.
4. Cai J, et al. Prog Retin Eye Res 2000 Mar;19(2):205-221.
5. Giblin FJ. J Ocul Pharmacol Ther 2000 Apr;16(2):121-135.
6. Deguine V, et al. Pathol Biol (Paris) 1997 Apr;45(4):321-330.
7. Dillon J. Doc Ophthalmol 1994;88(3-4):339-344.
8. Makashova NV, et al. Vestn Oftalmol 1999 Sep;115(5):3-4.
9. Taylor A, et al. Free Radic Biol Med 1987;3(6):371-377.
10. Beatty S, et al. Br J Ophthalmol 1999;83:867-877 (July).
11. Green K. Ophthalmic Res 1995;2727:143-149.
12. Ravalico G, et al. Invest Ophthalmol Vis Sci 1996 Dec;37(13):2645-2650.
13. Harris A, et al. Arch Ophthalmol 2000 Aug;118(8):1076-1080.
14. Groh MJ, et al. Ophthalmology 1996 Mar;103(3):529-534.
15. Mares-Perlman JA, et al. Arch Ophthalmol 2000 Nov;118(11):1556-1563.
16. Brown L, et al. Am J Clin Nutr 1999 Oct;70(4):517-524.
17. Ritch R. Curr Opin Ophthalmol 2000 Apr;11(2):78-84.
18. Popova ZS, et al. Vestn Oftalmol 1996 Jan;112(1):4-6.
19. Delcourt C, et al. Arch Ophthalmol 1999 Oct;117(10):1384-1390.
20. Babizhayev MA, et al. Peptides 2001 Jun;22(6):979-994.
21. Ferris, F et al. Arch Opthalmol 2001;119:1417-1436.
22. Sommerburg O, et al. Br J Ophthalmol 1998;82:907-910 (August).

When shopping for a good eye formula supplement, look for these ingredients to give you the full benefits of clear, sharp vision:

Vitamin A (as natural mixed carotenoids from D. Salina	3,500-4,000 IU
Vitamin C Ascorbates (corn-free)	200-400 mg
Lutein	15-20 mg
Vitamin E with mixed tocopherols and tocotrienols	200-400 mg
Zeaxanthin (from marigold)	3-5 mg
Astaxanthin	.4 mg
Bioflavonoids	300 mg
Bilberry leaf, (25% anthocyanosides)	120 mg
Taurine	600 mg
L-Glutathione	20-40 mg
Alpha Lipoic Acid	200 mg

N-Acetyl-L-Cysteine…………………………………………	200-400 mg
Eyebright herb……………………………………………..	50-70 mg
Grape seed extract (95% anthocyanosides)………………	100-200 mg
Ginkgo biloba leaf dry extract, 25% ginkgo Flavones glycosides, 6% terpene lactones……………………….	80-120 mg
Zinc polynicotate…………………………………………..	15-20mg
CoQ10……………………………………………………	100mg twice daily
Carnosine…………………………………………………	500mg cap
Omega-3 Fish Oil (mericury-free)………………………..	3-6 daily
Black Currant Extract (New Zealand)………	One 300mg cap, once daily
Curcumin (Turmeric Spice Extract): Helps reduce cataracts, diabetes, arthritis, bowel diseases, cancer, inflammation (Mercola.com)…..	2 daily

Dr. Rudi Moerck reports that scientific lab testing has shown Black Currant Extract to have specific anthocyanins that boost blood flow to the eyes and deter hydrogen peroxide oxidation. Currants have high antioxidant levels for increasing healthy vision; it also contains natural vitamin C.

We hope you have enjoyed reading Perfect Eyesight, as much as we enjoyed writing it. We challenge you now to take the next step in your quest for improved vision. That next step is practical application. Any achievement in life requires **practice, persistence** and **consistency.** Natural eyesight training requires the same dedication and discipline as any other goal in life. Dr. Bates said, "Eyesight is your most precious possession." You cannot afford to lose it. Others' have perfected their vision, and so can you. Start on your vision training program today, with just a few minutes daily, and enjoy the blessings of **Perfect Eyesight** for the rest of your long healthy life!

Write, email or call us if you have any questions, or tell us of your progress in improving your vision. We would like to hear testimonials from people around the world who have benefited from the teachings presented in **Perfect Eyesight.** Best wishes and blessings in your quest for Perfect Eyesight and super health.

For more information or if you would like an Appointment for Eyesight Training, Nutritional Body Typing Analysis, Deep Tissue Massage Therapy, Tai Yoga Massage or Chi Kung Energy Training Call:

HEALTH FORCE RESEARCH CENTER
Robert Lewanski, aka R.T. Lewis, Natural Eye Trainer,
Health, Diet, Weight-Loss and Nutritional Body Typing Coach,
Chi Kung Tai Yoga Shiatsu Massage Therapist
Chi Kung Instructor, Personal Fitness Trainer
2222 Hempstead Dr.
Troy, MI 48083
248-680-8688

Website: www.healthforcecenter.com   Email: healthforcecenter@gmail.com

References

Bates, William H., MD., Perfect Sight Without Glasses, New ,York City,Central FixationPublishing Co., 1920

Chaney, Earlyne, The Eyes Have It, York Beach, Maine, Samuel Weiser, Inc., 1987, Chia, Mantak, Chi Self Massage, Huntington, New York, Healing Tao Books, 1986

GMZ Productions Inc., The Eye Improvement System, Home Video, New York Corbett, Margaret D., Help Yourself to Better Sight, New York: Prentice-Hall, Inc., 1949

Gvoquan, Yang, Three-Bath Qi Gong, Hong Kong: Hai Feng Publishing Co., LTD, 989

Leviton, Richard, Better Vision in Thirty Days, Boca Raton, Fl., Globe Communications Corp., 1994

Peppard, Harold M., Sight Without Glasses, Garden City, New York, Blue Ribbon Books, Inc., 1940

Revien, Leon, OD. and Gabor, Mark, Sports-Vision, New York: Workman Publishing, 1981

Richardson, Dr. R.A., Strong Healthy Eyes Without Glasses, Kansas City, Missouri, Eyesight and Health Association Publishers, 1925

Rofidal, Jean, DO-IN: Eastern Massage and Yoga Techniques, Wellingborough, Northamptonshier, England, Thorson Publishers Limited, 1981

Ross, Dr. John R. and Rehner, Dr. Lowell, The Complete Eye Exercises for the Strengthening and Correction of Defective Eyesight, Plymouth, MI, Hall Publishing Company, 1943

Rotte, Joanna, Ph.D. and Yamamoto, Koji, Vision: A Holistic Guide to Healing the Eyesight, Tokyo: Japan Publications, Inc., 1986

Svoboda, Robert E, Prakruti: Your Ayurvedic Constitution, Albuquerque, New Mexico, Geocom Limited, 1988

Vision WorkOut, Inc., Vision Workout, Home Video, Reno, Nevada

Shaftsbury, Edmund, Instantaneous Personal Magnetism, Meriden, Conn, Ralston University Press, 1926

Appendix A
Source Page
Order Product List

Eyesight Improvement Training DVD – New Release!

Eye Healing Techniques and Eye Exercise DVD
NEW SHORT VERSION EYE IMPROVEMENT EXERCISES 15 -MIINUTE ROUTINE
by Robert Zuraw, Master Eyesight Improvement Trainer
Send $15.00 plus $3.00 shipping & handling

Chinese & Indian Yoga Masters of the Orient have practiced these Eye techniques to prevent eye disorders and to keep good eyesight far into advanced age. In this informative, inspiring DVD you will be shown, step-by-step, how to improve your vision using these same ancient healing secrets.

Audio CD – New Release!
The Secrets Behind Perfect Eyesight – Perfect Eye Habits

Discover the Secrets of How to Improve Your Vision Naturally! Find out the habits that weaken vision, & the Natural Habits that Strengthen Vision. $10.00 + $2.00

An inspiring audio CD on Visual Education. Thirty-Five years of practice, research, experience and wisdom on achieving clear sharp vision. If you want to get your natural vision back, this is for you.

To Order the "Perfect Eyesight" Book

1. Eyesight Improvement DVD. NEW RELEASE, Short Version, R. Zuraw, $15 + $3
2. Perfect Eyesight Radio Interview with Robert Zuraw on www.thepowerhour.com, with Joyce Riley, (www.gcnlive.com)--CD Audio $8 + $2
3. Oriental Secrets of Health & Healing, with Robert Zuraw DVD© - $10 + $2
4. Inner Secrets of Spiritual Wisdom, Harmony/Peace, Robert Zuraw CD© - $10+2
3. Secrets Behind Perfect Eyesight: Perfect Eye Habits. Audio CD - $10 + $2
4. Perfect Eyesight Book – $24.95 + $4 shipping
5. Pinhole Eye Exercise Glasses - $19.95 + $3 shipping
8. Chinese Five Element Nutritional Body Typing Energy Analysis Chart, one-time, life-time Consultation fee: $175.00

Make Checks or Money Orders payable to:
Robert Lewanski
2222 Hempstead Dr., Troy, MI 48083, 248-680-8688.
Email: healthforcecenter@gmail.com
Website: healthforcecenter.com

All products can be ordered from website and paid through **PAY PAL**
For quantity bulk BOOK discount orders go to Amazon.com, book orders

Appendix B

IN MEMORIUM OF ROBERT ZURAW

A Great Spiritual Warrior, Robert Zuraw, Master Eyesight Improvement Trainer, and Co-Author of the Perfect Eyesight Book Passes into the Light
A Spiritual Message of Help and Hope for Humanity
By Robert Lewanski, January 29, 2007
Co-Author of Perfect Eyesight

I have decided to tell the whole story of the life and teachings of Robert Zuraw, so that the new reader of Perfect Eyesight will know without doubt what kind of man he was. He was not a writer. That was my task. Robert Zuraw was a philosopher, an inspirational guide, teacher—a friend to anyone who needed help and a shoulder to weep on. He never gave up hope, even near the end, just before the diagnosis of liver and colon cancer—a few days later his body left the planet, and his spirit soared. Here then is the story of help and hope to all who will live this message.

Robert Zuraw was born on November 9, 1941 at 9:30am and passed into the Light on December 14, 2006, after years of quietly suffering from Agent Orange poisoning, while in Saigon, Viet Nam for 2 years, as a Medical Operating Room Field Hospital Nurse. He was a Staff Sergeant. This field Hospital was a similar operation as depicted on the M*A*S*H tv series in the 70s. He was under heavy Agent Orange spraying for 2 solid years, debilitated with 2 years of diarrhea and sickness while stationed there. (Agent Orange never leaves the body, and its half –life in the environment is 300 years!). Bob knew and studied about spiritual principles, and while stationed in the war zone, he "consciously raised his level of spiritual consciousness" to a higher level of love and peace, and protection for all those around him. In his immediate unit, for 2 years, no one was ever hurt or killed. He expressed the power of high spiritual consciousness and love, and it expressed itself as protection and peace surrounding the Medical Army Base. With all the toxic spraying, guns and bombs exploding all around him, it is a miracle that he made it out of there alive! But Robert Zuraw did survive and made it out of the "hell zone." And to survive another 43 years gives testament to his dedication and practice of the natural health and healing principles that most of us take for granted.

Because he was kind, considerate and put other people first, he stood up with bold courage, against a tyrannical Army General and Colonel Surgeon on the Army Hospital Base, protecting other, more defenseless South Vietnamese workers and lower ranking army staff.

When he came out of Viet Nam in 1964, he was very ill, and could barely walk. He went to see a Russian Herbalist in Windsor, Canada for herbs to detox the Agent Orange and heal himself. The herbs helped tremendously. He then studied and embarked on a Cleansing Detox Diet, eating only a raw fruit and vegetable diet for 40 days, similar to the Gerson Therapy Cancer Diet, he felt great and full of energy. The book he studied was entitled "Diet of Oxygen." Out-of-print now.

However, in the mid-80's, he had another set-back of dizziness and liver weakness, and was helped by Korean Zen-Taoist Master, Hynoong Sunim, with herbs and diet. He felt better soon after. Then again in the mid-90's the Agent Orange came back on him—and he went on another detox diet program. In mid-2005 he began having intuition and premonitions that he would be ill again. And, this time, in the Summer of 2006, he started to feel his liver hardening up, and he developed colon problems and diarrhea. In mid-December 2006 he was diagnosed with terminal liver and colon cancer; finally having constant diarrhea and loss of kidney function, and he could not stand up or walk. The ambulance came on December 8, and took him to Emergency room at Troy Beaumont Hospital. Two days in intensive care, and less than one day in hospice at Beaumont, and he passed into the Light In 2004 he weighed 187 lbs, and slowly lost weight down to 135, and on his passing 100 lbs. He was 65.

On December 13, at 5pm, he told me he was seeing Angels and Guides coming in and out of his third eye center, and that he would be well taken care of, and not to worry about anything down here on earth. In the early morning, at 2:15 am of December 14, 2006. Robert Zuraw passed into the Light, without pain, without medication and peacefully and quietly, just as he lived.

In spite of the Agent Orange chemical poisoning from Viet Nam, Robert Zuraw still managed to improve his vision from advanced progressive myopia 20-600 vision to 20-20 vision over several years of discovery, learning and much eye training practice. He kept his good vision right up until the end.

A Memorial service was held at the Theosophical Society on Woodward in Berkeley on January 28 at 1pm. We thank the staff at the Theosophical Society for offering their building for the Memorial Service. The building was packed with 80 of Robert Zuraw's closest friends. Everyone there acknowledged that he indeed embraced and lived the teachings of the "Three Treasures of the Tao or God-- the Way of Heavenly Light." The first Treasure is to be kind; the second is to be simple; and the third is to not put one's own importance fist in the world. Master Hua-Ching Ni says thusly: "Because kindness and compassion can produce courage, and simplicity can thus be broadened to contain the world. By not putting your own importance first…you will not impede the natural growth of all things. Kindness will invite the corresponding energy of kindness from Heaven through all the divine beings who support and protect." This is how Robert Zuraw lived his life, and all present at the Memorial agreed that he set a good Heavenly example for all of us to follow. Robert never complained, or told anyone about his health problems. Right up until the end he had hope of overcoming his liver and colon cancer, but it was not in the cards this time, and his spirit "left the temple-body," to merge with the Creative Light Energy of the Universe.

On the night of his passing a beautiful Meteor Shower passed over the northern hemisphere above the hospital. And the sages say that this is a good omen of an achieved spirit passing into the light.

We wrote three books together: "Ancient Secrets of Health and Long Life," "Health Force,"(typeset by Cindy Saul and PhenomeNEWS staff in 1982), and "Perfect Eyesight." (New revised edition 2011). Robert Zuraw's eyesight was perfect right up the last week of his life, and he was seeing clients for eye training 3 weeks before passing. I will carry our work of eyesight training, Chi Kung, Nutritional Body Typing, lecturing and workshops, and writing other books on Chinese and Ayurvedic Medicine. The following is a positive Channeled Spirit message from Robert Zuraw, through……

Theresa Miller Channels Robert Zuraw's Message of Hope and Peace to Humanity

Medical Intuitive, psychic and Channeler, Theresa Miller went into deep trance meditation and Robert Zuraw came to her with this message: "Tell Robert Lewanski. and friends that I have never felt better. Tell everyone that I see things so clearly now. I didn't really need to make my father be the scapegoat for my own self-doubt anymore. I see now that humanity creates all of it's OWN suffering—there really isn't anything wrong, ANYWHERE! Suffering is all a self-created illusion. We are all co-creating our beliefs of separation and then playing them out, over and over, in a dance of illusion--you know what I mean. I have decided that I am only going to participate in the NEW Earth, this is the one not yet manifested by most of the conscious humans yet--but it is coming! MAN, is it COMING!!!

You have no idea how incredibly beautiful it is in the spirit world! The Earth is surviving, my dear friend! Humanity is waking up to LOVE and its true beauty! I'm telling you, I can see it! I am going to be participating with that experience—don't worry, it's coming. By 2020, total world peace for all!

ALL of your world leaders will sign a pact to ERRADICATE war completely. It's already happened, my brothers and sisters. I can see it now and in the future!!! It's so beautiful! So, be of good cheer, keep sending the LOVE around the world, and trust and know that everyone's fears are being healed now.

It's really all going to be so wonderful!! Trust it!! I am doing great--I feel SO amazing! I love you all, and know that GREAT THINGS are coming! I can see them!" Theresa says in conclusion: "I can feel how happy he is, he really is ecstatic. He's really at a high spiritual level. THAT IS SO COOL!!! I can so clearly hear how life goes on in his spiritual energy. He's really happy."

Perfect Eyesight

And the Good News is Still Coming In

Robert Zuraw is having fun in the Heavenly realm now as reported below:

Two psychics said Robert Zuraw's Spirit was coming and going from the house here in Troy, to higher spiritual world--traveling a lot now—something he never did much on earth. He is having fun now. Psychic Intuitive, Paula Marie called earlier with condolences, and said Robert Zuraw was right here while I was talking with her, then all of a sudden he took off to the Higher Realms. She said Robert was a little angry with himself, but not in a hurtful way, more in a playful spirit kind of way, for leaving the planet so early, and not listening to my good advice about going for more help earlier. Anyway, another Medical Intuitive, Monica Levin said part of Robert is here, and part of him is in the spirit world. And Psychic Predictor, Michelle Stemmer said Robert is happy and enjoying his Mom and relatives in the higher spirit realms.

So, apparently, he has gone thru the lower planes of the astral realms, and ascended like a Taoist Immortal, and can come and go throughout the universe. That is good news for all of us to look forward to. We are all happy for him, and release him to the Immortal Realm of the Creative Universe or God (Tao). He beat the odds from Viet Nam, and lived 43 years fairly healthy. He had a wonderful peaceful life and will be missed by all who knew him, with all his wisdom, love and kindness. On behalf of all his students, clients and friends, we salute the life of Robert Zuraw and wish him a happy journey to the Light of immortal Freedom.

Robert Zuraw was the premier Natural Eyesight Trainer in the nation, and he had 20/20 vision, even a few weeks before his passing at age 65! He was a Scorpio-Metal Snake. I wrote the Perfect Eyesight book with him. He has helped and inspired thousands of people to better vision without glasses or contacts.
.
Robert Zuraw's valuable Natural Eyesight teachings will continue to be spread across the globe with my help and the help of our good friends

I thank all of you for your spiritual support, condolences and love.

Love and blessings to all of you,
Robert Lewanski
January 1, 2007

APPENDIX C

The Science of Earthing:
Grounding to the Earth is a Vital Key to Improve Your Health and Heal Your Body and Eyesight

We have all been taken away from the healing energies of the earth. The earth produces healing negative ionic electricity. It produces "FREE ELECTRONS" that we all need to heal and keep us healthy. All animals in nature are naturally grounded or "earthed." The new term for this ancient practice of barefoot walking is called "EARTHING,' from the book "EARTHING: The Most Important Health Discovery ever?" Published in 2010, this amazing book, written by Clint Ober, who discovered the principles of Earthing or Grounding, and co-authored by Dr. Stephen T. Sinatra and Martin Zucker.

Earthing covers over 10 years of testing, double blind placebo research in clinicsand universities and hundreds of testimonials, attesting to the power of Earthing or Grounding the body, either by barefoot walking on grass, beach or cement, or by using simple grounding devices or pads and bed sheets attached by copper wire to a ground rod outside, or to the ground circuit of your house electric outlet plug.

Testimonials are coming in by the thousands, from people who are using these Grounding Pads while sleeping, at their computers or in cars. The earth is the most powerful source of natural healing energy that comes into your body as "free electrons," which is healing energy to all animal life on earth. The authors say that we are "electrical beings on an electrical planet." The earth heals if we let it do its job, by walking barefoot, or using a grounding device, which bring the earth's healing energies, via the ground rod, to a conductive pad on your body, right inside your own home. Grounding can improve vision.

Most people are now "Electron Deficient." If you have pain, inflammation and illness, you are lacking sufficient electrons to heal your body. We are living in an Inflammation Nation, because we are not plugged into the earth on a daily basis. We wear rubber or synthetic shoes, live in homes with synthetic floors, ride in care with rubber tires, work in highly toxic Positive EMF high-rise building and work with computers and environmentally damaging electronics, including cell phones and laptops.

Barefoot walking or Grounding devices can also improve your vision, as the free electrons come up from the earth through your feet or a grounding device, and bring healing energy to your brain and eyes. Go to www.youtube.com and watch videos on Earthing and Grounding by Dr. Stephen Sinatra, David Wolfe and Clint Ober. Read the book, "Earthing: The Greatest Health Discovery Ever? (Ober, Sinatra, Zuckerk, 2010). Also, read articles on double-blind clinical and university science studies behind the Earthing phenomenon at www.earthinginstitute.net or earthing.com. YouTube "Longevity Now Conference." Your life will take on new meaning. Happy Earthing!

APPENDIX D
Your Personal Health Coach and Nutritional Energy Consultant
Rebuild Your Health with Correct Foods That Match Your Personal Internal Body Type Energy

The Most Comprehensive Nutritional Body Typing, Health, Nutrition and Energy Analysis System Ever Developed—The Ancient Chinese Taoist Four Pillars Five Element Personal Energy and Health Analysis Body Typing System and Ayurvedic Nutritional Body Typing Wisdom

"Within you is your own unique genetic code that unlocks the secrets to, and matches your individual body type. Unlock this secret code, and you discover your key to perfect health." It's simple when you have the key, and profound when you see and feel your body, health and life regenerate before your eyes!

Private Coaching Session with Robert T. Lewanski aka: R.T. Lewis
This unique opportunity will change your life

R.T. Lewis is a passionate Certified Nutritional Coach who makes wholistic health and healing remarkably simple and practical. He can put the pieces of your health and well-being puzzle in the right order for you. Born with a unique capacity to understand, apply and practice wholistic health and healing, Robert has a unique, caring and direct teaching method. His style and depth are a trinity of whole mind-body-spirit healing wisdom researched from the 5,000 year old Chinese and Ayurvedic medical systems, to the latest modern research into healing on the DNA and chromosome telomere level, healing with breath, breakthrough supplements, and accessing healing from original essence or spirit. He has the ability to take profound wholistic health and healing teachings and break them down into practical daily wisdom. You can understand and apply something better in a creative, positive manner, when it is taught in an easy to understand way. Health and energy benefits can come quickly, without all the hocus pocus, guess-work and side-effects of just taking pills or drugs.

During your Private Coaching Session, you will discover your specific Body Type, what foods match your system, finding the core issues, and true causes of your health problem, and to get your health and energy zooming to a high level. Integrating his 40 years of experience, insights and perspectives, will save you years of poor health and time. The phone calls and emails can lead you toward a greater vision for your health and life. After the order is processed, Robert will email you for your personal appointment.

You'll Discover How to Eat Right for Your Individual Body Type System

Stop the guesswork of what you should eat to make you zoom, using the breakthrough science of Individualized Body Typing Testing. Get a genetically-correct, metabolically-balanced diet, herbs and supplement program specifically designed to maximize your energy, fat loss, health and well being. Comprehend and grasp the cause of your illness and guard your health and immune system through specific diet, herbs, breathing, exercises and mind habits.

The Most Precise System for Analyzing Your Body Type
This Oriental Nutritional Energy Analysis System
Balances Your Health and Five Organs for a Lifetime

☯Glandular Body Typing and Profiling.   ☯Ayurvedic Body Typing Medicine and evaluation of the 3 main body humors: Vata(Air), Pitta(Fire), and Kapha(Water). ☯Chinese 4 Pillars, 5 Element Constitutional Body Typing System.   ☯Oriental Diagnosis of sign and symptoms of health and disease   ☯In-depth Body Typing Evaluation Form

Discover Your Healing Health Medicine Within

Discover how the correct foods for your individual system can heal you, and how the incorrect foods can make you ill. Eating a "healthy well-balanced diet" without knowing your specific Body Type and glandular system can lead to poor health, fatigue and ill health symptoms. Are you feeding your illness and symptoms or are you strengthening your health, energy and life? Your healing medicine within gently guides you on the road to good health & well-being. Without good health, high energy and vitality, everything else you do in life seems meaningless. Take action today! Send for your Personal Evaluation, and I'll help you attain your health goals.

Your Personal Body Typing/Testing/Profiling Consultation

☯Stop PMS, cramps, prostate problems, diabetes safely and easily
☯Restore digestive fire and stop bloating, indigestion and poor food absorbtion
☯Lower cholesterol easily and safely, by eating these whole foods and supplements
☯Lower blood pressure and hypertension naturally, without toxic drugs
☯Lose weight safely, without cravings and swinging like a yoyo with your weight
☯Overcome fatigue, anxiety, moods, sugar cravings, yeast or candida infections
☯Blood building and foods the detox and cleanse your organs, liver and colon
☯How the 5 Element food tastes, seasons affect, your mind, health & emotions.

In this remarkable Eat Right for Your Individual Body Type System,™ you'll discover why some foods are healing medicine for you, creating good health and energy, and why other foods are a poison for you, creating weakness and disease. Find out why some foods are good for you, but detrimental to someone else? How would you like to solve this diet-riddle once and for all?

Can you have a lifetime of perfect health? Is there such a thing as diet freedom. The answer is a positive YES! If you are sincerely interested in discovering the real solutions and secrets of internal health and healing, preventing pain, suffering and illness, and regain your health, than you are in for a pleasant surprise. We all have distinct needs. No two body chemistries, energies, emotions, strengths, weaknesses A food requirements are alike. *Our bodies are unique, so no single nutrition program works for all!*

The Perfect Diet for You!

"You wouldn't downhill ski blindfolded, with your hands tied behind your back, would you?—so why are you doing it with your diet, which is supposed to sustain your life with good health and energy?"

Find Out How to Take the "DIE" out of "DIE-T"

A health profile is conducted. You are guided to the correct foods, herbs, supplements and exercises that match your individual body type system. Your glandular system is evaluated to determine food sensitivities. Weak and strong organs are found. Health problems & energy leaks are evaluated accurately.

With over 35 years of research, constant study and practice in the holistic health field—nutrition, herbs, exercise, chi kung, massage, oriental diagnosis, I can help you to regain your health, prevent disease and lose or gain weight back to normal. Discover why everything you've tried so far hasn't worked. This is the most important health secret you will ever discover about yourself!

Individualized Nutritional Body Type Diet Energy Analysis Charts
Five Element Four Pillars I-Ching Chinese Medicine and India's Ayurvedic Health Wisdom

The Chinese Four Pillars, Five Element Birth Chart Analysis

This Oriental Four Pillars Birth Chart is based on the energies that came into your body at birth, and formed your Physical Constitution from Heavenly Energies and Earthly Energies.

How soon can you see a difference in your health. Many people feel and see the benefits to their physical, mental and emotional health in one week. Others' take a little longer. When you feel a change for the better, you'll see how imperative it is for you to eat in harmony with your own Personal Body Type Character. You were born with your Specific Body Character, and it stays with you for a lifetime. You can keep it in good balance, or not—it is up to you. One complete Body Type Analysis is all you need to find out the healing foods you need to eat that will always balance your system and give you unlimited health and well-being. For a one-time, lifetime fee of $175.00, you'll have unlimited coaching, consulting and advice for as long as you need it to attain good health and energy balance.

In your analysis of yourself, include: health problems, complaints, symptoms, body weight, height, how long you've had the problem, health habits, exercise routine or lack of one, vitamin/mineral/herbs supplements you are currently taking, how much liquids/water you are taking in daily, where you may be carrying weight, i.e., upper, middle or lower body. Sleep habits, insomnia. Fatigue syndromes. Candida yeast infections, bad menstrual cramps...etc.. You get the idea! I will also send you through email attachment, an Ayurvedic Body Typing Evaluation Form to find out what single or dual Ayurvedic Body Type you are.

SYSTEMIC HEALING FORMULAS

You will have access to the most powerful healing formulas in the world. These special Systemic Healing Formulas are available through Certified Health Practitioners. These bio-energetic herbal tissue, gland and hormone healing RNA/DNA formulas were developed by the genius Master Herbalist/Nutritional Scientist, Dr. Stu Wheelwright, which is now carried on by his son Stu Wheelwright Jr., and passed on through the writings of Dr. Jack Tips at www.apple-a-daypress.com, who wrote about Dr. Wheelwright in "The Pro-Vita! Plan," "Your Liver, Your Lifeline," "New Dimensions in Herbal Healing," "Conquer Candida," "Greater Energy," and others. These Formulas are listed as "*Bio-Command Formulas*:" (Increases restorative action, enhanced assimilation, tissue receptivity and directs the combined herbal matrix toward specific cellular functions or commands). "*Bio-Function Formulas:*" (Nutritivet and therapeutic herbal combinations 'tuned" to specific tissue bio-energetic resonance matrix to support specific organs, body systems, biochemically and bio-energetically to optimize function and performance to restore body to good health). "*Bio-Nutriment Formulas*:" (Bio-available vitamin, mineral, essential fatty acids, friendly flora to maintain health, e.g. herbal chelators for B-Vitamins, multi-bio-nutrients for optimum assimilation that take these formulas to a higher level of restoring health and vitality). "*Bio-Extract Formulas*:" (Special formulated oils and liquids that help heal external conditions and internal immune challenges). "*Concentrated Extract Formulas*:" (Liquid extracts which are rapidly assimilated for quick results and health benefits). "*Bio-Pathic Formulas*:" (Homeopathic remedies to support the body's subtle energies). "*Bio-Challenge Formulas*:" (Formulas for nutrition for rebuilding, restructuring, environmental pollution, pathogens). "*Bio-Basic Formulas*:" (Nutritional support for internal bio-terrain, e.g., ACCELL for healing triad of (Digestion, Intestines, Liver), and ENZEE formula with special bio-enzymes to clean the extra-cellular matrix)."*Dragon-Rising Five-Element Formulas*:" (Constitutional formulas from Japan, China, South America, Indian Ayurvedic Herbs, combined with Western herbal nutrition to support body, mind and spirit healing). (Herbal formulas are available, and are additional to the basic lifetime consultation fee). Systemic Herbal Formulas will be recommended according to your constitution, health challenges, symptoms and needs, and they are rotated within these formulas to bring about complete health, healing and well-being.

Lifetime, One-Time Life-Time Consultation Fee: $175.00

For more information on Workshops, Seminars and Private Training for Perfect Eyesight Improvement, Chi Kung Yoga Energy Exercises, Chi Kung Tai Yoga Barefoot Shiatsu/Acupressure Massage, Nutrition and Health Life Coaching; plus, Herbal Therapy, Whole Food Supplements, Whole Food Recipes and Food Prep Classes, see contact information above.

For an in depth explanation of how this system works go to: **healthforcecenter.com**
Obtain Your Personal Chinese Five Element
Body Type Chart Through the Mail
Send your Birth Date: Year, Month, Day, Time and Location of Birth to:

Robert Lewanski, aka: R.T. Lewis
**Certified Ayurvedic Nutritional-Health Coach
and Practitioner of the Five Element Four Pillars Chinese Medicine
2222 Hempstead Dr. Troy, MI 48083
or call for an in-personal consultation: 248-680-8688**

e-mail: healthforcecenter@gmail.com   website: www.healthforcecenter.com

Perfect Eyesight

Appendix E

The Amazing Pinhole Eye Glasses!

If you suffer from **myopia** (nearsightedness), hyperopia (far-ightedness), presbyopia, astigmatism, computer vision syndrome, or cataracts—then you could benefit from **myopia pinhole glasses**. **How Pinhole Glasses Work**: Conventional Pin Hole lenses are made from opaque plastic material with small pinholes in the material. **Figure 1**, below, is a schematic representation of a bundle of light rays coming from an object in front of a myopic (nearsighted) eye. Improper refraction, or "bending", of the outermost rays (dotted lines) in that bundle of light by the eye is a cause of refractive errors such as myopia, hyperopia (farsightedness), presbyopia (diminished focusing range with age) and astigmatism. Pin Hole glasses can bring about clearer vision in all these conditions. These holes have the effect of reducing the width of the bundle of diverging rays (called a "pencil of light") coming from each point on the viewed object. Normally, the full opening of the pupil admits light. It is the improper bending of the outermost rays in that pencil of light which causes refractive errors such as myopia, hyperopia (farsightedness), presbyopia (diminished focusing range with age) and astigmatism to be noticeable. Pinholes can bring about clearer vision in all these conditions. By blocking these peripheral rays, and only letting into the eye those rays which pass through the central portion of the pupil, any refractive error in the lens or cornea is not noticed as much. The pupil may be wide open, but only the central portion is receiving light. The improvement in visual acuity can be dramatic.

Referring to the figure and the representation of a pinhole in front of the eye: by the lens blocking the outermost rays and allowing only the central rays (solid lines) to pass into the eye, a refractive error in the eye's lens or cornea is not as pronounced. In other words, the eye's pupil may be wide open, but only its central portion is receiving light. The improvement in visual acuity in this case can be considerable. By looking through Pin Hole glasses, instead of squinting, peripheral rays are blocked from all sides. Farsighted people can easily read close work. Pinhole's can allow you to see at ALL **(Figure 1)** distances. Pinhole Glasses can benefit people with cataracts, as they help focus the

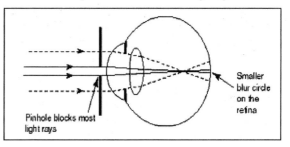

light without scattering the light. Pinhole Glasses can help you concentrate on details better, which improves visual acuity. :Pinhole Glasses take some getting used to. You'll see a "honeycomb effect" as you look through the holes. If you have a small refractive error or weak prescription glasses, you'll see easily through the holes with clarity.

Strong prescription eyes will take some getting used to. Over 6 diopters of nearsightedness may not be able to see with Pinholes. **Never** use Pinhole glasses while driving or walking, as peripheral vision is weaker; Pinholes are for reading, computer work or looking at TV, or at distance objects. Pinhole's also reduce sun glare and have built-in UV protection. They also reduce eye strain at computer monitors for long periods, causing fatigue, headaches, dry eyes, blurred vision and double vision.

How Pinhole Glasses Work

When you look at a blurred object your brain moves the focus of the eye in and out until it gets an increase in contrast. If no increase is achieved your brain leaves the object unfocused. Pinholes improve your clear sharp image, allowing your brain to find the point of focus. During this process the focusing muscles of the eye are getting used more and this regular exercise helps your eyes' focusing system to see clearly.   Figure 2

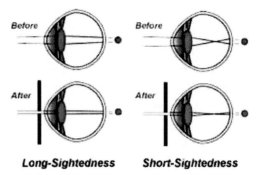

Look at this drawing, Figure 2, of a myopic eye with the rays that would need the most bending since they are blocked by the lens. It is said that Scheiner first described this effect in 1573. Those who are familiar with cameras will recognize that this is the same principle used to increase the depth of focus by decreasing the aperture. Pinhole cameras also operate by this principle.

One group that should not use pinholes, or any glasses that reduce accommodation (focusing effort), is young people who are very farsighted. These people need to accommodate as much as possible in order to reduce their farsightedness to a lower level. This is nature's dynamic method of refining visual acuity in the growing youngster and it should not be defeated.

Pinhole Glasses: Exercise your eyes while you read or watch TV. Farsighted people can do this exercise while focusing close up – doing things like reading. Near-sighted **people get the benefit from focusing at a distance, eg. Watching TV. The major cause of the long-sightedness that comes with advancing years is a weakening of the focusing muscles that control the eye's lens.** Looking through the tiny holes forces the eye muscles to exercise. **Just 15-20 minutes a day bring a noticeable improvement within a couple of weeks.**

Order your Pinhole Eye Glasses today: $19.95 plus 3.00 shipping.
Check or Money Order payable to: Robert Lewanski 2222 Hempstead Dr., Troy, MI 48083   Email: healthforcecenter@gmail.com.
Website: www.healthforcecenter.com. Call: 248-680-8688
Allow 5 to 7 days for personal checks to clear
Money Orders: Products will be sent promptly
Payments can also be made through PAY PAL on the above website

Appendix F
FAR INFRA-RED SAUNA TECHNOLOGY
By Phil Wilson – www.momentum98.com
RELAX Portable DETOX (Far Infra-Red(FIR) Light
Stands Heads and Shoulders above all other Saunas in effectiveness

We call The Relax Sauna the ONLY Portable Professional Model Sauna, since it is the ONLY Portable Sauna that we know of that generates 100% safe and absorbable Far Infrared Light. After 4 years of selling the Relax Sauna, we were shocked to discover that every other portable "FIR" sauna generates only about 30% far infrared Light. They use a far infrared cloth which covers a metallic grid, or hotplate. It appears that there is no legal definition of what a FIR Sauna is. When you see a sauna advertised as FIR, It means to me that it is at least 25% FIR Energy being generated. Each company "should" be able to tell you what percentage of the generated light is FIR light (healing light), which means the remaining generated light CANNOT be absorbed by your body. Most individuals selling these saunas have NO CLUE that their saunas are NOT even close to our 100% FIR.

On the other hand, our technology has been given a 510(k) number by the FDA, and it is regarded as a medical device. We use a patented semi-conductor chip to generate the healing FIR Light.

The FDA has also confirmed that the light generated by our radiators are guaranteed to be 100% absorbable FIR (healing) light between 4 and 14 microns. If you are considering getting another sauna for less money, we can assure you that their technology is primitive compared to the technology of the Relax Sauna. A paneled sauna using a piece of cloth, and a hotplate is probably only about 25% FIR Light.

Because it does not have intensity and purity, as does the Relax Sauna, it generally will not be as effective in terms of healing, and certainly will not feel as incredible as the Relax Sauna does.

In time, as we gather up testimonies, we will have these available to you, and each month, we expect to find those reading these pages will become convinced of the quality and effectiveness of the Relax Sauna. When We demo our sauna at Expos, we get lots of firsthand experience. Dozens of individuals who have not been using their expensive wooden saunas have purchased the Relax Sauna from us. (Their main complaint is that it takes too long to warm up). Similarly, scores of those who own other portable saunas have also purchased the Relax Sauna from us. (Their main complaint of other saunas' is that they don't sweat, don't feel THIS good, and that their ailments haven't been helped that much).

We have received a number of comments recently in the last few months by people who say they have done a lot of research and have concluded that the Relax Sauna is the Far Infrared Sauna that they feel is the most effective Sauna around, have purchased it from us, and are extremely pleased with the results that they are getting.

This is why more and more health centers, spas, healing centers, clinics, chiropractors, naturopathic doctors, acupuncturists, and massage therapists are choosing to use the Relax Saunas in their practices! Go to www.momentum98.com and read the testimonials and watch the videos on this amazing product. Only the Far Infrared waves between 4 and 14 microns can be absorbed by the human body.

Other saunas emit near Infrared, or Medium Infrared light which is resisted by the body. Its wavelengths are NOT in harmony with human energy. Ultra Violet energy is much stronger than near infrared, and because of this, our body resisting this energy causes friction, and as a result of this intense friction caused by the body's inability to absorb this light, can cause suntan and even sunburn.

The Healing Energy of Far Infrared Light sort of feels like a cross between enjoying a very nice warm shower, lying in a warm sun, and basking in the arms of, I guess you could say, Divine Love. Not very scientific, but, in Taiwan, they say that being in the Relax Sauna is like being in the presence of a Chi Gong Master—divinely tuned individual.

Suffice it to say, that being in the Relax Sauna really feels Wonderful! We believe this "HEALING LIGHT" helps get rid of anything that is Dark (dark moods, funky moods, depression, etc.), and anything that is heavy (heavy metals, fat, mucous, toxins etc.). After all, LIGHT is the opposite of darkness, and it is the opposite of heavy. And there is a reason they call it LIGHT.

Recent research has shown: Spending 15 minutes in the Relax Sauna is as good (or better) than a 45 minute cardiovascular workout, in terms of burning calories.

<u>Huge Diabetic Ulcer (1.5" x .75") clears in 7 weeks, 20 minutes per day</u>. This is a case study of a large diabetic ulcer that was healed using the FIR Professional Radiator. Doctors had not been able to do anything with it for 1 1/2 years. We show this information and pictures to nurses, and they are truly, truly amazed at what the Relax Far Infrared Ray Sauna can do. <u>Relax FIR Healing Case Study</u> (*287 KB pdf*)

<u>Smaller Diabetic Ulcers clear up in 2 months after Sauna treatments twice a week!</u> One lady who owns a spa in Philadelphia bought our sauna because she was impressed with this report. She has since reported to us that she has had two clients who have had maybe 5-10 diabetic ulcers on their legs. In both cases, the ulcers cleared up in 2 months, using the sauna just twice a week.

<u>People who have been in accidents are getting pain relief in minutes 1st time in 4 months!</u> In our store, we have had a number of people come in and go into the Relax Sauna for 5-10 minutes. One lady who had been in a rear ended car accident came in for a 10 minute treatment, and found such relief, she came back a week later with her sweats on, and spent 15 minutes in the Sauna. She cried after that, since she was able to be pain free for the first time in 4 months.

Another lady, a health professional, was just in the Sauna for 5-8 minutes. She called two weeks later and said that this was the only thing that has given her relief from an accident she had had, hurting her leg. So she had to get a Relax Sauna from us.

Massage Therapists have great results—their clients melt like butter! We have been having amazing reports recently by many health professionals, and massage therapists. We had a massage therapist in Detroit have such incredible success in 3 days after she got a Relax Sauna from us with one of her MS clients and others. She called us and told us that 3 of them wanted Saunas.

A special friend of mine who has been a massage therapist for about 6 years, has been telling her friends and other massage therapists that "You want to work smarter, not harder," as she explains to them, that after she puts her client in the sauna, she can do more good for her clients with a 20 minute massage than with a 55 minute massage with no sauna treatment. You'll get enhanced health benefits using both the sauna and the OXYOZ OZONE GENERATOR, the first comprehensive Ozone Oxygen Mini-Spa System for Air, Water, Shower, and Bath, from www.momentum98.com. (SEE APPENDIX J).

A massage therapists in the Columbus area got a Sauna from us, and relayed to me his experience. He said massaging people after they have been in the sauna for 10 minutes is like "putting butter into a microwave." They just melt, and he can do wonders. A lady in the Cincinnati area who does re-connective tissue work said to me, "Yes, for sure." Usually, she can do a 1 hour re-connective tissue work session in 20 minutes after her client has been in the sauna. The other day, she was able to complete the job in about 10 minutes.

Testimonial from Bob Lewanski, (aka R.T. Lewis), Director of the Health Force Research Center in Troy, Michigan, Deep Tissue Massage Therapist, Tai Yoga Massage Therapist, Chi Kung Practitioner and Instructor, Practitioner of Five Element, Four Pillars Chinese Medicine, Certified Ayurvedic Nutritional Counselor, and co-author of Perfect Eyesight: The Art of Improving Vision Naturally, says: "The Far Infrared Sauna is absolutely amazing in imparting health and energy and chi to the body. Before I see clients for massage, I get into the FIR Sauna for 30 minutes daily to get charged up with high level Chi

Energy and warmth. Then I am ready to work on massage clients in a relaxed and intuitive manner. I have clients get in the sauna for 20 minutes before a massage, and they are totally relaxed and loose after the Sauna. They just plop on the massage table, and because their muscles, joints and tendons are warm and flooded with FIR Chi energy, I can release stressed out areas of their body. The FIR Sauna does this like nothing I have ever tried. For even better results, use the Fir Sauna along with the Oxy/Oz Ozone Machine, (from www.momentum98.com), to get powerful Ozone into your cells, tissues, organs and brain. Both the FIR Sauna and Oxy/Oz machine help greatly to improve your overall immunity and boost your energy levels, and detox your entire body, right down to your cellular level and DNA. Use these two powerful health devices daily, at the same time, and you may quadruple your energy and health. Your personal chi energy will just zoom. May the Health Force be with you! Best of health and healing. Health Force Research Center, Troy, Mi, 248-680-8688. www.healthforcecenter.com

Dr. George Yu's (MD), Detoxification Protocol for Fat, Toxins, Chemicals, Drugs, Alcohol

Dr. George Yu, M.D. LIVE from The Longevity Now® Conference 2011, YouTube. Here is a body fat and chemical, drug Detox Protocol you can see on YouTube.com, with David Wolfe, and Dr. George Yu, M.D., at the Longevity Conference, California. Dr. Yu gives us this Protocol for cleansing the cells of fat and toxins: He says this Protocol "Explodes" the fat and toxins right out of the cells.

STEP 1: Take 100 to 200mg Niacin. You'll get a red itchy flush throughout your body, head and face—Dr. Yu says, "Get over it—that's part of going through this cleanse. The flush is secondary, the real flush is going on in your fat cells. STEP 2: Exercise or jump on a mini-trampoline for 20 minutes to get your lymphatic system stimulated to kick out fat and toxins. STEP 3: Immediately after your exercise, get into a FIR Sauna, regular sauna, or any type of heat source for 40 minutes, (to create sweating, which helps to remove fat and toxins from your cells and tissues. STEP 4: Take 5 capsules of _Food Grade Activated Charcoal,_ and 1 Tbls. _Calcium Bentonite Clay Powder_ (food grade). You can empty the charcoal capsules into a glass of water or juice, and mix together with the Bentonite Powder—drink immediately. Do this every day for a week. Or, you can do it on weekends, when you have some free time. This is a very powerful cleanse. Take extra magnesium citrate capsules—2 or 3—to keep your levels high, to replenish your cells after all the sweating. Eat plenty of raw fruits and vegetables during this Detox Protocol to increase your cellular fat and toxin removal. Take one or two lemons daily, squeezed in water. Eat grapefruit, oranges, pineapples, berries, green vegetable salads, herbal detox teas etc. When your body is clean and functioning optimally, your vision can also improve.

Saunas are $1,195 retail, and if you tell them you read it here, in Perfect Eyesight, you'll get at least $200 off retail price. This can be a great benefit for your overall health, detox, well-being, longevity and vision improvement.

"Please visit our health store in Clintonville, we would love to meet you!"
Phil Wilson - 3509 North High Street, Columbus, Ohio 43214
We're open 7 days a week! Hours: M-F:10-7, Sat:10-6, Sun: 12-6 EST
PHONE: 1-800-533-HERB (4372) & 614-262-7087 -EMAIL: moment98@gmail.com

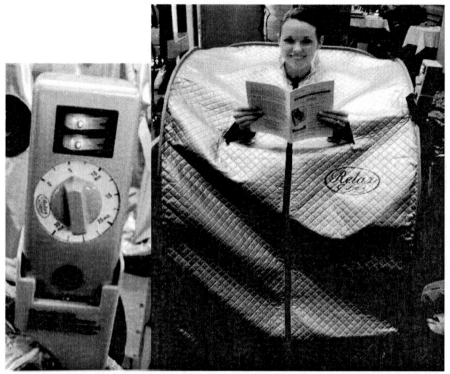

Timer Controller   Far Infrared FIR Sauna

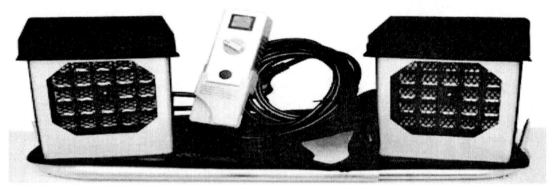

**Far Infrared Radiator with 40 Semi-Conductor Micro-Chips
(Shown with cord and Timer-Controller Switch)**

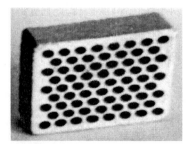

20, 1 inch Semi-Conductor Chips on each side—40 total

Appendix G
The Amazing Power of Cartenoids, Astaxanthin, Zeaxanthin, Lutein, Vitamin C—Plus, Mica Miracle— New Breakthrough Detox Liquid, for Health, Environmental Detox and Vision Improvement

Astaxanthin is a powerful carotenoid supplement. It is produced by ocean microalgae *Haematoccous pluvialis*. It is a free radical scavenger, like lycopene, lutein, beta-carotene and alpha-tocopherol, protecting cells, organs and tissues from oxidation. Astaxanthin is up to 65 times more powerful than these other carotenoids. It is 550 times more effective at protection from excessive sun exposure. Astaxanthin crosses the blood-retinal barrier to protect your vision— the others cannot make the cross-over. It protects DNA damage, and it reduces inflammation. You can't get enough Astaxanthin from food, like microalgae or fish. Supplemental form of 3 to 4 mg. is the best protection for your eyes. Carotenoids are pigments found in all colored vegetables—beets, carrots, spinach, raspberries etc. Carotenoids are important in the photosynthetic process and protect the plant or life form from light or oxygen damage. Carotenoids found in zeaxanthin, lutein, the gold color in chanterelle mushrooms astaxanthin contain oxygen; other carotenoids do not. Zeaxanthin is contained in corn, kiwi, grapes, orgnges, peppers and squash. Zeaxanthin is found in fresh, raw vegetables and fruit. You are not getting enough Astaxanthin from common foods—get it from pink salmon, which feed on plankton, which feed on microalgae, which make the Astaxanthin pigment. Wild salmon are 400 times higher in Astaxanthin than farm fish. Astaxanthin is amazing because it helps boost immunity, reduces C-Reactive Proteins (CRP, lowers triglycerides, and improves good HDL levels, boosting heart and artery health. Reduces cataracts, macular degeneration and blindness, improves brain function and lowers dementia and Alzheimer's, reduces many cancers; helps nerve cell damage, reduces inflammation of arthritis and asthma; improves endurance and recovery; it levels off blood sugar, which improves kidney function; reduces digestive and reflux problems; increases sperm; prevents sunburn and all kinds of radiation; helps pancreatitis, ms, carpal tunnel, arthritis, Parkinson's, Lou Gehrig's and neurological problems;

Why does Your Eyes Need Carotenoids?

Carrots are loaded with cartenoids (Vitamin A, or retinal) for clear vision in your retina. Blindness comes from lack of Vitamin A or Carotenoids. Zeaxanthin and lutein are contained in the retina, which is high in fatty acids, more than anywhere else in the body. The retina is a light and oxygen loaded area, so it requires these powerful anti-oxidant free radical scavengers, to keep the eyes healthy and prevent oxidation. Zeaxanthin and lutein are needed there in high concentrations for the vision to see clearly. The yellow color in the macula of your retina contains a "yellow spot," and is fed by these two pigments.

Zeaxanthin is concentrated in the central macular retinal (fovea), where much light converges for clear vision. That's why we need to eat a variety of colorful yellow, green, red, orange, purple fresh fruits and vegetables. Your vision simply needs these colorful food elements to perform optimally.

Macular Degeneration and Cataracts are the Leading Causes of Blindness
Astaxanthin is the best carotenoid to prevent blindness. Fifty million people go blind, over 50, from aging macular degeneration. And 20 million become blind from cataracts. Vitamin C, from Ascorbates (not ascorbic acid, which is made from high fructose corn syrup). Vitamin C, along with zeaxanthin and astaxanthin, work together to keep vision healthy and strong. Vitamin C cannot work along. Lutein and zeaxanthin reduce cataracts and macular degeneration, and increase the pigment density in the macula, which slows down the aging macula. I use all three of these carotenoids to keep my vision in tip-top shape. However, astaxanthin is the most potent free radical eater, and it easily crosses over the blood-brain-retina barrier, more than lutein or zeaxanthin.

Scientists, like Dr. Mark Tso, of the Wilmer Eye Institute at Johns Hopkins University, have studied lutein, zeaxanthin, canthaxanthin, and astaxanthin for their respective abilities to protect the retina. Astaxanthin is easily the winner in all studies. However, lutein and zeaxanthin assist and boost healthy vision, and make astaxanthin work better. All these carotenoids have no side effects to worry about. They are from whole foods, from ocean plants or herbs. Dr. Tso reported that astaxanthin can prevent macular degeneration, diabetic neuropathy, macular edema, glaucoma, all eye inflammations and more. Other scientists (Shimidzu et al, Bagchi, Martin et al, and Beutner have corroborated Dr. Tso's research on astaxanthin.

Astaxanthin Prevents Cancer, Supports Immune System in Animal Studies
Studies have shown "improved antitumor responses..."(Kurihara et al, 2002). Tanaka et al (1994), showed protection from urinary bladder cancer. In 2002, Kurihara et al studied the protective effect of astaxanthin against cancer in mice. He found astaxanthin "improved antitumor responses by inhibiting the lipid peroxidation induced by stress." He also found (1995) study in preventing oral cancer in rats. Beta-carotene tested good too, but astaxanthin even better. Same results with colon cancer—lessening incidence with the use of astaxanthin in lab animals. Wild pink salmon is high in essential fatty acids and astaxanthin. Astaxanthin can also help build immunity in elderly people, as shown in animal studies by Harumi Jyonouchi at the University of Minnesota.

For further research on astaxanthin, read "Astaxanthin and Cancer Chemoprevention" by John E. Dore, Ph.D of Cyanotech Corporation.

Author's Note: *With all this good research on eye supplements, you still need a whole food diet, healthy lifestyle habits, exercise, rest, sleep and low stress to make your life and health operate in a synergistic balanced way.*

Burn Fat and Rev-Up Muscle Endurance

Astaxanthin has also shown to boost muscle endurance and metabolize fat—it is a fat burner, combined with exercise, or course. It boosts the membrane of the mitochondria that fuels ATP energy production. Astaxanthin, or any other supplements won't work wholistically, if you don't also improve your over-all health, well-being and fitness levels.

Astaxanthin Contains Sunburn Protection Properties

Astaxanthin has also shown to protect from sunburn, by "singlet oxygen quenching". Take 2 mg daily for a 30-40 days, and you will not get sunburned easily. You won't see results if you pop astaxanthin just before going to the beach. It needs 4 to weeks to saturate into your cells and tissues. Of course, you don't want to lie in the sun in Cancun for hours, and expect not to burn. Common sense is sometimes not so "common." Astaxanthin is from ocean microalgae, which contains the same antioxidant power to protect itself from powerful sun rays—it does the same for you. If you schedule for an x-ray or CT scan, take 2-4 mg astaxanthin 4-6 weeks before the scan, and you'll have some protection from the radiation. Same goes for constant flyers and airport dwellers—never stop taking astaxanthin, and you'll have constant protection.

Do you want the best natural source of astaxanthin and omega-3 fatty acids—use krill oil. Get it from www.Mercola.com.

Along with 2-4mg of astaxanthin daily, eat a diet rich in fresh organic fruits, vegetables, soaked seeds, nuts, soaked whole grains, get enough exercise, good sleep, meditation, stretching or yoga and chi kung and above all, get "Earthed." Go to www.earthinginstitute.net or www.earthingyou.com, to get grounded, and let the free electrons coming from the earth heal your body and brain. All the best in your quest for super health and Perfect Eyesight! Thank you and be blessed. Also, do your deep breathing exercises daily, with your OxyOz Ozone Machine turned on.

Mica Miracle

Mica Miracle is the safer, better, cheaper, easier, and greener way to purify your water.

Mica Miracle makes. eliminates and denatures 99.9% of all toxins including:
*Germs *Mold *Fungi *Bacteria – like staph and E coli. Will purify pond, lake or pool water. It's like a water filter, a mineral water, and an electrolyte drink all in one!

Purifies and ionizes water of any quality. Just add 2 or 3 drops per glass of water or liquid.
* Delivers 70 trace minerals—including three of the rarest minerals on earth
* Enhances hydration by reducing the size and surface tension of water molecules

**Mica Miracle makes bad water good and good water great! Can help your overall health, vision and well-being, by reducing environmental pollution and metals in your body.
Mica Miracle $30.00, 3 fluid oz. Order from www.thepowerhour.com or call: 877-817-9829**

Appendix H
The Liver-Stomach-Colon Triad and Traditional Chinese Medicine (TCM) in Relation to Vision and Eyesight Health

Chinese medicine has known, for 8,000 years, that the liver controls and feeds the eyes and vision. If you have a headache around the eyes, you likely have a congested liver. Poor nutrition and weak energy and lack of blood flowing to the eyes, will cause fading vision, cataracts or macular degeneration. The health of your eyes is dependent on the health of your liver and digestive fluids, like bile coming from the gall bladder and liver.

The human body is a living Chi or energy producing biological organism, like all life forms on earth. When your liver, colon and other organs are weak, the eyes and vision become distorted with myopia, hyperopia, cataracts, glaucoma and macular degeneration. Chinese medicine see all eye problems as a liver and gall bladder problem. Liver acupuncture points are located around the eyes, and gall bladder points are on the side of head above the ears. Acupuncture for the liver improves vision, as well as massaging all the points around the eye arch and side of the head, as discussed in the Chapter on Dao-Yin Massage.

The liver can regenerate itself, even at 30-40% functioning. It will come back if you eat the right foods and supplements, and bring the Chi healing energy back into your liver and body. You have to give it the right conditions through healthy diet, exercise, supplements, rest, Earthing or barefoot walking or with indoor Earthing pad devices. **(See Appendix C).**

Glaucoma and cataracts occur because the small blood vessels inside the eye get congested with atherosclerosis, from a diet too high in animal fats, animal proteins, simple sugars, white flour carbs, smoking, alcohol, excess oils, especially rancid, or trans-fat oils, like commercial soy, corn, canola (mustard seed/rape seed oil).

To strengthen your liver, avoid eating 3 hours before bed, so the liver can rest and heal properly, without over working to digest food during the night rest cycle. Sour foods strengthen the liver, i.e., lemon, grapefruit, plum, sauerkraut, pickles, sourdough bread, all used in moderation. Try this: In the morning drink (squeeze) one lemon in a glass of warm water or herbal tea—this cleanses and strengthens the liver, and improves your true appetite and hunger.

Overeating and junk food is the greatest cause of weak vision. Eat to ½ or ¾ full and stop. Overeating pushes and twists the internal organs out of shape. Go for a slow walk after eating for 15 to 20 minutes—this helps digestion and allows the blood to stay in the stomach for thorough assimilation, absorption and elimination to take place naturally. Close work directly after meals weakens digestion and vision, because the blood goes to the head, instead of the stomach, which eventually causes many health and eye problems. **To improve liver and eye function, eat these foods:** Raw and steamed vegetables, sprouts, soaked seeds and nuts, green, leafy vegetables, spinach, black sesame seeds, parsley, soaked almonds and sunflower seeds, carrots, broccoli, beets, Brussels sprouts, raspberries, blueberries, cherries, and fresh figs. If you wants to avoid eye and health problems, avoid these foods: fried foods, refined white flour products, sugar, fruit juices, dairy products, coffee, chocolate, alcohol. If you want to eat meat, eggs or poultry, get the farm raised organic kind, and keep them down to 5-10% of your total diet. The human body requires about 70-75% vegetables cooked and raw, 10% fruit, 10-15% protein, 20-40% whole grains and root vegetables, 5% seeds or nuts. If you want fish, obtain wild caught fish, like cod, white fish, salmon, a couple times a week. If you have blurry vision and are light sensitive, go on a liver cleanse. The liver is the life-line to your health, perfect eyesight and longevity. Take care of your liver, and it will take care of you!

Detox your Liver, Colon and Stomach to Improve Your Vision

If you want clear sharp vision, you need to keep your liver squeaky clean. The liver is the major body cleanser and detoxifying organ. It filters out poisons from drugs, environment, alcohol, water, environment. It also filters out excess fat, cholesterol, artificial flavors, preservatives, toxic water and processed chemicalized foods. Your liver saves you from dying on a daily basis. When the liver is overloaded with excesses of all kinds, toxic wastes then accumulate in the liver, organs, tissues, cells and blood—this is called "toxemia" or toxic overload, and this is the major cause of "dis-ease", or un-easiness in your body, mind and spirit. There is only one cause of most diseases—that is toxemia, which is developed by two pathways; 1) malnutrition, and 2) toxic excessive acid overload in the cells, tissues and organs of the body. When this occurs, the body develops a multitude of disease symptoms stemming from the colon, stomach and liver. If you clean up these three organs, your body will heal itself naturally. But, you have to give it the right organic whole foods, enzymes, probiotics and supplements. The liver is amazing; it can regenerate, even if 2/3 of it is damaged or diseased, when you go on a detox program to detox the liver, colon and stomach of undigested and toxic debris. Smoking, marijuana, alcohol, drugs, chemicals, heavy metals, polluted air, environmental toxins are also major causes of liver breakdown.

When the liver is not operating optimally, it is congested with free radical toxins or scar tissue, which causes oxidation of tissues. All forms of pollutants, alcohol, cigarettes, fluoride in water, sugar, excess fats of all kinds, drugs, cocaine, heroin, marijuana, all create free radical damage, and cause scarring inside the liver. When your liver goes down, so does your vision and eye health. High fat foods, beyond the liver's ability to metabolism them, is converted from fatty acids to low-density lipoproteins (LDLs) and high-density lipoproteins (HDLs) in the liver. Too much fat in the diet makes the liver overwork, and it can't do its job of filtering out the normal toxins on a daily basis.

Here is how to regenerate your liver: Eat a diet high in antioxidants and low in fat, preservatives and chemicals, and your liver will regenerate itself. High beta carotene foods, green foods, green super powders with vegetables and fruits, carrots, raspberries, acai berry, pomegranates, blueberries, vitamin C ascorbates, Vitamin E Mixed tocotrienols, astaxanthin, lutein, zeaxanthin and quercetin.

In the Chinese Five Element System, the liver is damaged by anger, and if a person is angry continually, the liver further weakens, and vision gets blurry and fuzzy, and the eyes become red with furry. Anger stops blood circulation to the liver, heart, lymph and liver, which cause chi or energy stagnation in the liver, causing more congestion and disease. Calmness and kindness heals the liver. The Chinese liver healing sound is "ssshhhh." Take a deep breath and exhale the sound "ssshhh" through your teeth and rounded lips. Kindness and calmness help to improve vision and healthy eyes.

Other whole foods for the liver are: sprouted wheat bread or wheat sprouts or wheat grass. Wheat increases circulation inside the liver, produced liver chi or energy, and help toxin removal from within the liver. Eat lima beans, green beans, split peas, leafy greens, spinach, broccoli, parsley, collards, all high in fiber and antioxidants to keep the liver and eyes healthy and strong. Carrot, celery and beet juice cleanse and detox the liver, and are rich in antioxidants. Eat all kinds of seaweeds, like kelp, dulce, arame, kombu etc—rich in minerals, and vitamins A and B, and boosts internal immunity. Squash is rich in beta-carotene and antioxidants. Fermented foods like, miso, tempeh, sauerkraut, pickle, pickled beets, strengthen the intestinal tract and help the liver to function optimally. Wheat germ (toasted) contains good Vitamin E. Spirulina and chlorella are rich in protein and antioxidants.

Garlic protects the liver from cancer causing agents. Sunflower, broccoli, alfalfa and mung bean sprouts contain life-giving oxygen and chlorophyll. Sweet rice, made with the herb mugwort, helps strengthen the liver. Brown rice vinegar sprinkled on a bowl of fresh garden vegetables feeds the liver and promotes clear vision. Sour foods enhance liver function, ie., grapefruit, lemon, limes, granny smith apples, sour cherries, sour oranges, sauerkraut. Herbs to enhance liver and impart clear eyesight: Celandine, culler's root, goldenseal, milk thistle, burdock root, dandelion, beta-carotene supplement, vitamin E—400 IU (mixed tocotrienols and tocophorols daily), N-Acytel-Cystiene (NAC), glutathione, selenium (yeast bound), Vitamin C ascorbates, astaxanthin, lutein, zexanthin.

In excess, the following foods weaken the liver and cause poor vision: Keep these foods low in your diet, (or eliminate them altogether if you can, or at least eat organic free-range foods, and eat no more than 5%-10% of total diet): eggs, red meat, milk, cheese, peanut butter, nut butters, nuts—unless you soak them overnight. (nuts, grains and beans have enzyme inhibitors and phytates in them, which bind up minerals in the body and cause digestive problems in many people). All nuts, seeds, grains and beans must be soaked overnight in water to reduce digestive, absorption and assimilation problems people have with eating these foods. Alcohol excess causes liver disease. One-half glass daily will not harm you, but act as a tonic, especially if it is produced organically, without sulfites and pesticides. **Disease causing products:** White flour, pizza, drugs, marijuana, cocaine, heroin, coffee, soft drinks, sugar, fruit juice (unless diluted by ¾ with water), white rice, white bread, low fiber noodles, packaged, processed foods and fast foods, and frozen processed "foods." Avoid these foods, and your health and vision with zoom!

Chinese Medicine the Liver-Eye Connection and the Liver Flush Program

If you have a **weak liver or deficient liver,** heat symptoms may appear, i.e., red tongue and face, little thirst, hot hands and feet, insomnia, possible irritability, depression, nervousness and dry, hot-inflamed itchy eyes, blurry vision and poor close and distant vision. A congested hot liver can easily form gall stones in the gall bladder, as the liver and gall bladder work together to produce good health and vision. If **stones or sediment form in the gall bladder,** you could have these symptoms: indigestion, gas, pain in upper right rib cage, tightness in upper shoulder/neck area, bitter taste, chest pain and blurry vision. If you have many of these symptoms, you need a **Liver/Gall Bladder Cleanse/Flush:** Eat lots of raw and streamed vegetables, blueberries, raspberries, apples, especially Granny Smith apples, one or two lemons and grapefruit daily. Do this for at least a weak. Then, on the morning of the eighth day, eat only apples throughout the day—4 to 6—helps to soften the gall stones. Also, drink some green juices, and herbal teas including ginger, cinnamon, bilberry, boldo, dandelion, eyebright, artichoke leaf, barberry, Oregon grape root, peppermint and yellow dock. You can get some of these herbal bulk teas at Whole Foods Market or online. Before bed, warm up 2/3 cup of organic olive oil to body temperature, and stir together with 1/3 cup lemon juice. Sip slowly, and go to bed. Lie on your right side, with right leg pulled up to allow the gall bladder to pass stones in the morning. If you can't do this flush, just eat the salads and a variety of vegetables, and pour 2-3 tablespoons of olive oil and lemon juice on the veggies. Do this 2 or 3 times per day. Eat the fruit separate from the vegetable meal. Many people have avoided gall bladder surgery and improved their health and vision with this amazing **Gall Bladder Flush/Cleanse Program.**

Eat these herbs, spices and foods to decongest and heal your liver: watercress, onions, mustard greens turmeric, basil, bay leaf, cardamom, marjoram, cumin, fennel, dill, ginger, black pepper, horseradish, rosemary, all mints, lemon balm angelica root, prickly ash bark. Go easy on the hot peppers, as they can make the liver hotter and cause stagnancy. **Liver detox foods:** beets, taro root, sweet rice, amasake, straw berry, peach, cherry, chestnut, pine nut, cabbage, turnip root, kohlrabi, cauliflower, broccoli and Brussels sprouts. Sprouted wheat, rye, buckwheat, seeds, fresh raw and steamed vegetables and fruits. Small amounts of honey and apple cider vinegar are powerful liver detoxers. Other helpful herbs to heal the liver out if its stagnancy: romaine lettuce, asparagus, amaranth, quinoa, alfalfa, radish leaves, citrus peel, bupleurum, Mandarin(chai hu),chaparral, milk thistle seeds, chamomile, peony, peppermint. To cool the liver: mung beans, mung bean sprouts, celery, seaweeds, kelp, dulse, cucumber, tempeh (soy fermented protein food), millet, plum, mushrooms, rhubarb, red radish and white diakon radish. To further boost liver healing, eat spirulina, wild blue-green algae, chlorella and wheat grass. Kale, collards, chard, alfalfa are excellent liver cleansers and healers.

The liver and vision become weak from over-eating animal foods, like beef, chicken, eggs, dairy, pork, butter, cheese, milk, which create stagnant heat and wind conditions inside the body. Keep these foods down to 5-10% of your total diet, and your health, energy and vision will improve dramatically. Plus, stop eating sugar, sweets, white flour, cakes, pies, pizza, drugs, marijuana, smoking etc. You and only you can heal your body and vision. Perfect Eyesight can be yours if you follow this program consistently.

New Dimensions in Herbal Healing for Healthy Vision

A revolutionary system of using herbs bio-energetically, by herbal researcher, Dr. Stu Wheelwright, who made amazing and revolutionary breakthroughs in natural healing and herbology, including: 1) "herbal polarization principles, 2) tissue frequency (bio-energetic) compatibility, 3) solutions to many of herbal medicine's limitations, and 4) the pinnacle of his 40 years of research—the **6 Systemic Bio-Command Formulas.** Proper application of the Wheelwright Healing System "provides the clinician and {practitioner}, an unprecedented degree of precision and comprehensiveness in herbal/nutritional therapies that produces faster, more thorough, and more consistent remedial results." (New Dimensions in Herbal Healing, Dr. Jack Tips, 2003). One such formula that helps improve eye health and vision is the **#50 I-(Eyes).** This formula "relieves eye stress, eyestrain, supports the optic center (back lobes) of brain, nourishes clear vision." Good for close work, computers, diabetics, helps prevent diabetic retinopathy. Formula I-(Eye) supplies natural vitamins and 13 other eye factors to give nutrients to help strengthen eye muscles and tissues associated with good vision." This formula can be used in conjunction with other Systemic Nervine Formulas to help vision: **B (Brain Formula), N (Nerve Formula), Nc (Calm Formula), and N3 (Relaxa Formula).** You can get all these formulas at www.apple-a-daypress.com or call 24 hours a day: 1-877-442-7753 or 1-800-445-4647. To further your understanding of how the liver heals the body, read "Your Liver…Your Lifeline (Healing Triad)," and the Pro-Vita Plan, by Dr. Jack Tips.

Appendix I

The 20 Secret Physical, Mental and Spiritual Keys to Good Health and Long Life ©2011 Perfect Eyesight by R.T. Lewis

1. **EAT ONLY WHEN TRULY HUNGRY**. True hunger is present when your mouth waters, sensation of hunger in throat, (which makes mouth water) and tongue is pink and clear. A coated white, yellow or dark tongue indicates internal intestinal or stomach is stagnant with previous undigested food matter. Food digests properly when you are happy and relaxed, and true hunger is present, which makes your inner digestive juices, enzymes, pepsin, hydrochloric acid come alive. When food digest well, there is no bloating, gas or fatigue after meals. When digestion is smooth, your body and organs function healthfully, emotions are smooth, and spiritual-intuitive sensitivity expands and you become successful in all your goals. Overeating is indulging in sensual mind appetite—causing body illness, spiritual insensitivity, pain and suffering, and a short unhappy life. East Indian Ayurvedic Medicine stated over 5,000 years ago that "There is no disease, without first, gastrointestinal derangement." This is the first and most vital Key to Health and Longevity. If food does not digest properly, the liver and vision will weaken, and eye diseases can develop.

2. **PROPER ACID/ALKALINE & YIN/YANG BALANCE.** Depending upon your health condition, in warm or hot weather, eat 50%-80% raw vegetables, 10%-15% fruit, and 20-40% cooked foods. Cold weather is yin. Hot weather is yang. During cold winter weather, eat more cooked soups, whole grains, beans, casseroles, and protein foods, to keep warm and good internal balance. Eat with the seasonal changes and you will maintain your acid/alkaline pH balance. Eat 60-80% steamed, sautéed, broiled, baked foods in cold yin weather, and 20-30% raw foods—salads, some fruit etc. Pay attention to how you feel, & what you require on a daily and seasonal basis. If you get cold easy, or have cold hands and feet, stay away from cold raw food in winter, and have your thyroid checked for hypo- or under-activity; also, avoid raw cabbage family vegetables, like raw broccoli, cabbage, Brussels sprouts, kale, chard, collards, bok choy, which can create goiter and a weak thyroid gland. You get more nutritional value from these cruciferous vegetables steamed on the soft side. If you are a hot Pitta or Lesser Yang Hot body type, you can eat more yin raw fruits and vegetables and feel good. (See **Chapter Seven**: A Complete Protocol and Analysis of Nutritional Body Types…). (See also **Appendix D**, Nutritional Body Typing Consultations and Systemic Healing Formulas to balance your internal glands and organs).

3. **EAT ONLY WHOLE NATURAL FOODS MOSTLY.** Choose whole sprouted grains cooked: wheat, brown rice, millet, oats, corn, buckwheat, barley, quinoa, amaranth and rye. Eat fresh organic chemical-free vegetables and fruits, seeds and nuts. Avoid processed and preserved foods. If you eat fish, get the wild caught Alaskan fish. If you are a Vegan food eater, choose non-GMO organic foods. If you eat meat, keep it down to 5% to 10% of diet and use only organic pasture raised or free range chicken and eggs. Keep animal foods low, and you will avoid cancer and attain health and longevity. Use Sea Vegetables (kelp, dulse, arame, kombo, hijiki—which are rich in minerals and boosts immunity, health and longevity, and helps reduce weight. Natural whole foods improve vision and eye health.

4. **CHEW FOOD WELL.** Your stomach has no teeth! Chewing well brings out the sweet taste in foods. When sick fast 1 to 5 days, or eat only vegetables, stews, soups or rice. Whole food complex carbohydrate (vegetables, whole unprocessed grains, seeds, nuts, legumes) digestion starts in the mouth with the saliva enzyme Ptylin, which converts food into nutrients usable by the body. Animal foods do not require a lot of ptylin for digestion, mainly hydrochloric acid in the stomach. Chewing develops spirituality and sensitivity. Mental clarity and good judgment improves with mastication, and leads to satisfaction after eating, and minimizes overeating. Fast eating creates stomach, colon and small intestine diseases, which reduces health, well-being and longevity. Poor digestion further weakens eye health and vision.

5. **NEVER EAT IN PAIN, TIRED OR IN EMOTIONAL DISTRESS.** These states cause body enervation or fatigue, and impedes digestive juices, which causes indigestion. As stated in #1 above, when you do not have real true hunger, and eat anyway, internal undigested food toxins will accumulate in the

stomach, colon and liver "The Triad of Health." Read, "Your Liver, Your Lifeline" by Dr. Jack Tips. Eat when relaxed and cheerful. Wait until you are calm and rested. If you are tired and upset do not eat, or take some warm herbal tea or soup. To eat when emotionally upset or fatigued creates poor health, poor vision and a short life. When tired, emotionally distressed or in pain, rest or sleep or seek help from a holistic health care practitioner.

6. AVOID HOT & COLD FOOD AND LIQUIDS. This suspends digestive fluids and wastes body energy. Eat food warm, but not too hot or too cold. Avoid iced drinks before, during and after meals as this suspends paralyzes digestive enzymes and secretions. Also, avoid drinking before, during or after meals, as this waters down the digestive fluids (pepsin, hydrochloric acid, enzymes), and can cause gas, stomach upsets, diarrhea and other gastrointestinal derangements. Wait 2 hours after eating to take liquids, or 1 hour before solid foods. Extreme cold or hot foods can cause a mucous buildup, as a reaction in the body, to the extreme temperatures, which can further cause digestive problems, weak vision and poor health.

7. FASTING OR CLEANSING DIETS . Water fasts, lemon juice cleansing program, raw fruits and vegetables, and their juices are all good body cell, organ and blood cleansers when the body requires it. Best time is during warmer Spring or Summer weather, when fruits and vegetables are in abundance. Overeating is the greatest cause of disease, poor health and weak vision, as it taxes the liver, colon and stomach organs, creating congestion and internal organ derangement. Periodically eating lighter cleansing foods, herbal teas, fruits and vegetables, reduces internal toxins and cleanses the colon, liver and stomach of undigested stagnant foods. When in doubt, rest, fast and sleep until true hunger returns.

8. PROPER FOOD COMBINING. Incompatibility in foods can cause gastric upsets in some people. Avoid raw fruits with any cooked carbohydrates or protein. Eat raw fruit on an empty stomach, especially melons. All fruit digests quickly, (15 minutes), and if eaten with other foods, can cause gas, bloating and indigestion, because they ferment, while the other foods digest first. Acid raw fruits can be combined with proteins, like lemon or pineapple with fish or nuts/seeds or nut milk. Generally, eat raw fruit alone, or leave it alone. Fruit can be cooked, as in apple pie, and eaten separate from the main meal, and will not cause indigestion. Whole grains are combined with any raw or cooked vegetables, stews, soups, casseroles or beans. Protein foods combine well with raw and cooked vegetables. Pure protein foods, like meat, fish, eggs, combine poorly with any carbohydrate foods, like grains, bread, potatoes.

9. EAT ONLY TO 80% STOMACH CAPACITY. Stop before full. Overeating causes excess diseases—more is taken in than eliminated. Overeating brings excessive blood to the lower digestive system to help the digestive process, and takes blood away from the brain. Overeating causes weak stomach acids and retards digestive enzymes, bile, pancreatin and pepsin. Mental clarity is diminished with a full stomach. If your stomach is constantly full, especially with junk food, your brain and memory can become foggy, weak and forgetful. An alert clear mind equals success, inner security, good health, vision and longevity. Excess eating, beyond what the body requires, is a sure road to illness and a short life. Benjamin Franklin once stated: "Lessen your meals to lengthen your life." Lab animals fed a calorie restricted diet, lived 3 or 4 times longer than the overfed lab animals.

10. ENJOY YOUR FOOD. Eat with the spirit of thankfulness, gratitude and enjoyment. Prepare food with natural ingredients, with health and good natural taste in mind. Use natural mild spices and herbs to enhance the taste of various dishes. If natural whole foods don't taste good, you won't eat them. Herbs, spices, sauces, dips and dressings properly prepared can ad zest and variation to your whole foods recipes. Be mindful of what you eat, when you eat and where you eat. Enjoy meals with family and friends.

11. THE KITCHEN IS YOUR NATURAL HEALTH PHARMACY. Your daily food is your internal medicine. Choose whole foods wisely; proper preparation of daily meals is crucial to well-being. Most illnesses are avoided with proper nutrition. No need for doctors if you eat healthy, organic, non-GMO foods; develop good insight, study and research into your personal body type, natural food recipes, menus, hot and cold weather conditions, personal health condition, rest, sleep, stress and emotional states. "Physician, heal thyself," can be applied to your kitchen food pharmacy and how you use it on a daily basis.

12 BODY, EARTH, AND SPIRIT NOT THREE: Your body is not separate from heaven and earth. We are all ONE with Great Nature. It is an incorrect attitude to think we are separate from this earth or the heavenly realm. To enhance physical sensitivity and spiritual cultivation, eat more vegetable quality foods. Lessen animal foods, dairy and refined sugar of all kinds, including excessive juices. These foods can weaken your ability to feel, heal and diagnosis other's diseased conditions or poor health. Eating whole natural foods increases awareness that we and the earth are One Integrated Whole. Our understanding and sensitivity to others will increase dramatically, with clarity and wisdom. Let go of non-creative thoughts and you'll increase your health, energy and longevity. Practice positive, creative affirmations daily.

13. GO OUTDOORS AFTER MEALS AND AVOID CLOSE WORK. This practice can improve your health and longevity dramatically. Why? Oxygen helps to digest food. Indoor close work--reading, tv, or computer work after eating a meal causes poor digestion, because the majority of blood, required for digestion is drawn into the brain, head and eyes, and not enough blood stays in the stomach to facilitate proper food digestion.   This weakens vision, because the poorly digested food creates internal undigested food toxins, that circulate to the brain, head and eyes, causing poor eyesight, headaches and possible brain fog or memory loss over time. Take a few deep breaths while walking and gently swing your arms to and fro—this increases digestion and heart and lung circulation throughout the body. When food is not digested properly, because of too much close work after meals, poor health and poor vision are not far behind. Walk at least 30 minutes after meals and look softly into the distance. This one practice, according to Dr. Sasaki, a eye doctor from Ann Arbor, MI can add 20 to 30 healthy years to your life. Even a 15 minute walk after meals can do wonders for your digestion and overall health and longevity. Barefoot waking on clean grass or the beach improves health, vision and longevity and proven in scientific studies. (See **Appendix C:** Earthing/Grounding Barefoot Technology for Health).

14. NEVER EAT A HEAVY MEAL BEFORE BED TIME. This is a big no-no if you want good health, mental clarity and to keep slim and trim. Eating at night puts on weight for Kapha (Water) types, and causes mental sluggishness in all people. Night hours after 8pm are for healing and rejuvenation of cells, tissues and organs, not for ingesting heavy proteins and other foods. Eat your last meal before sunset if possible, or at least 3 or 4 hours before sleep. Sleeplessness is caused mostly from overeating late or overdrinking liquids all day, which weakens the kidneys and liver. When food is forced to digest late in the evening, the internal organs, i.e., liver, stomach and kidneys become over-active and won't allow your brain to produce serotonin and melatonin, which allows your brain to turn off and go into a natural sleep cycle. Tossing and turning is a sure sign of the internal organs trying to digest and process foods. And they won't let you sleep when they are working hard to digest what you ate late at night before bed. If you are starving late at night, have a piece or two of whole grain bread or an apple to take off the edge of hunger. You will sleep soundly, and wake up with natural hunger, without the grogginess or sluggishness caused by late night heavy dinners.

15. EXERCISE DAILY. Our bodies were made to move each day. Walking 2-4 miles a day is good. Walk in the woods. Walk by a lake or ocean. Walk in the mountains. Walk in the city, or walk at the Mall on cold icy days. Walk with a friends or a group, or walk alone.   But, WALK. Take a yoga class. Get a massage, perform chi kung movements. Use light weights and squatting exercises for body tone. Swing your arms to and fro vigorously daily for heart and lung circulation.   Do some stretching Yoga daily alone or with others. Chi Kung, and Tai Chi are good energy conducting movements for health and longevity. If you don't move and breathe deeply every day, you get stiff and old in body, mind and spirit. Move it or lose it!

16. DRINK PURE LIQUIDS WHEN THIRSTY ONLY. No animal in nature drinks when they are not thirsty. If you eat enough vegetables, grains and fruit (whole foods), your thirst will be normal. Over-drinking is the cause of much kidney, bladder, colon and stomach problems.   Water is not an inert substance. Water can cause water-logging of the entire body if taken to excess. The man who wrote the book on drinking more water, died of a water disease—water on the lungs—pneumonia! Heed the warning, and drink when you have real thirst. If you are sweating a lot in the hot sun, take more water, but add a few drops of trace minerals from sea water, and purchase Electro-Mix by Alacer Corp to put electrolytes in your water before drinking. Also, ad Willard Water (Catalyst Altered Water CAW), a few drops to each a glass of water—this hydrates the water for better assimilation and cellular hydration, so you don't need to over-hydrate and bloat your cells and tissues with excessive non-hydrated liquids. (**See Chapter 7,** sub-heading at end of Kapha Body Typing Analysis: **"How Much Water do we Really Need?"**)

17. REST OR SLEEP WHEN FATIGUED OR EXHAUSTED. When your body and mind are tired, rest. Nature is telling you to rest or sleep when you are tired or sleepy. When you are fatigued or exhausted , mentally and physically, lie down and rest or sleep. Proper rest and sleep rejuvenates your kidneys and adrenals, your longevity organs, which regenerate your life force. Your body knows best and gives you signals daily. If you do not heed the signals—you create more stress, fatigue, tiredness, headaches, exhaustion, anger, impatience, frustration and nerve depletion—you'll end up in an emergency room or nut house! Slow down, take ten deep breaths, go outside and walk barefoot in the grass or beach. You'll avoid a nervous breakdown, and improve your health and energy; and, perhaps, get to play with your great great-grandchildren. Go to this excellent website: www.earthinginstitute.net, for grounding and earthing wisdom and grounding devices.

18. MODERATION IN ALL THINGS. Taoist, Zen, Buddhist, Christian Mystics and Yoga teachings all say to avoid extremes. "Extremes" cause extreme diseased (inflammation-fever conditions in the internal organs, muscles, and cause body/mind/spirit imbalances, leading to suffering and illness. Live a simple, joyous life. The real key to a healthy physical, mental, emotional and spiritual life is to live in harmony and balance with people, nature and heaven. Imbalance is a terrible disease, and leads to frustration, anger, worry, anxiety, fear, grief, hate, impatience, loss, mental illness, unhappiness, anguish and darkness. All your goals can be accomplished through practicing moderation and calmness. Rushing around with excessive ambition and anxiety only shortens your health and life force. Extreme activity leads to exhaustion, which exhausts your adrenals and kidneys—considered longevity organs in Traditional Five Element Chinese Medicine. When your kidneys and adrenals are completely burned out, your spirit and life force leave your body—you expire. So, protect your kidney system and you will preserve your health and reach robust longevity.

19. PRACTICE LOVE, KINDNESS, FORGIVENESS, THANKFULNESS AND GRATEFULNESS AT ALL TIMES.
Live in the **Now moment** as you move through your daily activities, & all your wishes will be realized. You express love, because the nature of creation is love, and you are creation. Be kind to others, and they will return kindness to you. If you give out negative emotions, you get back negative emotions from others. The creative universe is like an echo chamber; whatever you give out, you get back 10 times over. Before falling asleep, forgive others and yourself for all trespasses, big or small, and you'll sleep like a baby, and heal your life. Forgive those who oppose you. Be thankful for who you are, and for everything in your life—thank the trees for giving you oxygen, the oceans for healing ions, the sun for growing your food and healing your body; thank your family and friends, and thank the Creative Life Force for giving you a healthy body to express all these positive emotions. Be grateful for every little thing that comes your way—for your food, for your wonderful home, for an opportunity to serve and help others in need. If you are grateful, the Creative Universe will be grateful to you, and allow you to realize your every wish!

20. CULTIVATE YOUR SPIRITUAL ENERGY. PRACTICE CLEANINESS OF BODY & MIND. Keep your work space clean and uncluttered. Clean up after yourself, even if living alone. This is good Feng Shui, or order and neatness in your surroundings. Too much clutter, clutters your mind, spirit and emotions. Practice daily meditation. Sit straight in a comfortable chair and relax your entire body. Take very slow deep breaths in as your belly rises, and out as your belly moves in. Calm your mind, and dwell on the Light of Creation that flows throughout your body. Feel the light of heavenly energy circulating through your body. Relax and completely let go of all anxiety, worry, frustration, anger—just be with your breath, with an empty mind. If thoughts come, let them flow out. Just relax and release your life into the Creative Power that brought you here. "The kingdom of heaven is within," and "Be still, know that I AM."

Final Note: These are the Secret Keys to bring you good health and longevity. Practice them as best as you can. No one is perfect all the time, but practice helps you improve the health and healing of your body, mind, emotions and spirit. Refer to these 20 Keys often, and you'll eventually achieve superb health and disease-free longevity. So be it. Live long and prosper! Stay in the Light always.

APPENDIX J
The Healing Power of the Breath of Life Through Oxygen, Ozone and the OxyOz Ozone Generator

The ancient masters taught that the Breath of Life is the Breath of Creation, infused into life on earth. You can live with food for several weeks, without water for a few days, and a minute without oxygen. We take oxygen and breathing for granted. We know nothing of the amazing healing power of the pure oxygen that flows through the tiny air sacs of our lungs. Life is a miracle of breathing. The end products of digestion are the ash left on the lungs through breathing. Digestion is a respiratory process. We live and die by the breath or lack of it. When you discover how to get the Breath of Life into your lungs, brain, cells, tissues and DNA, at that moment, you will start living as a new Being.

Oxygen combines with iron in the hemoglobin as oxyhemoglobin. Ozone increases this process in the body cells. In illness, more oxygen is required. Disease is caused by lack of oxygen in the cells and DNA—the cells corrode or rust from lack of this Breath of Life—Oxygen. Lack of oxygen does not aerate the blood properly, so acidic wastes build up in the tissues, and the blood becomes anemic or deficient. This results from poor food choices, internal toxemia and poor internal and external respiration and transportation of body fluids. Inflammation is a lack of oxygen in the body. Oxygen is the Key Element for health and longevity. Low cellular oxygen results in physical degeneration and calcification (hardening), of tissues, organs, cells and bones. Ozone is the answer, as it breaks up and forms a stable molecular oxygen. If you need more oxygen to heal or to boost your energy, ozone is your answer. Ozone Therapy, in clinical use, reduces both acute and chronic inflammatory conditions, and arthritic calcifications. Ozone is used in hospitals and to sterilize water systems. Ozone is 1/5 as heavy as oxygen, as it moves up to higher regions, like mountains. The ancient masters knew this, and lived in higher regions with ozonated prana or chi to perform their immortal breathing cultivations. They live, even today, long and healthy lives in this pure ozone atmosphere, and they are in-touch with the higher and finer forces of the universe. The Yoga Masters of the Himalayan mountains and the Chinese Taoist Immortals live in the mountain dwellings in China. The mountains air has greater ionization than the lowlands and coastal cities, which are filled with smog and carbon monoxide. Ionization means "ions" in the air, which are electrified particles. Scientists have found that the atoms of the air gases, i.e., nitrogen, oxygen, ozone, carbon dioxide, are not "electrified" in their whole state. They get electrified when ultra-violet rays, cosmic rays, radium, x-rays, and electrons crush the atoms—the broken atoms turn into "ions" or electrified particles. People living in higher regions live longer because of this highly charged ozone and electrified ions. They experience a natural electrical rechargement, regeneration and revitalization of their cells and DNA. The more ozonated air you breathe in, the less food you need to live, and your health zooms.

Prana and Chi or Ki is not merely cosmic rays from the stratosphere, but more powerful ionized minerals and nitrogen that flow down from Cosmic regions, which is transformed into protein in the body, thus the body requires less dense protein foods. In the high ozone mountains, you breathe deeper and harder, because you come from the "lowlands" with low ozone. Low ozone means shallow breathing in low altitudes—so most of us become shallow breathers by the dense air of stuffy cities. Lungs never fully develop, and millions of air sacs in your lungs stay inactive and dormant. Ozone makes you breathe deeper, longer and stronger, and thus makes you live longer and healthier. Ozonated air is thinner air, so you have to breathe deeper to supply your body oxygen needs. You eventually get stronger and healthier, slimmer, trimmer, because you are getting more pure ozonated minerals and protein from the pranic electrified air. Your lungs become activated, as millions of dormant air cells in the deep areas of your lungs come out of their dormancy and become active, as they were meant to be. High elevations require time to adjust to the "thinner" ozone air, but when you do adjust, your health and vitality zooms way beyond the "lowland" city dwellers. You become regenerated with the pure ozone in high regions. Your lungs gradually expand, and your health improves at the same time.

Breathing Ozonated air is a respiratory process, that improves lung capacity, which also brings aerobic oxygen into your colon and digestive system. When the colon is congested with anaerobic (no oxygen), your lungs and respiratory also become weak or diseased. In Chinese Five Element Medicine, the Lungs and Colon work in unison. If the lungs take in poor quality polluted air, along with lack of deep breathing, and acidic junk food, the colon also becomes deranged from this lack of oxygen. On the other hand, when the entire gastrointestinal tract is congested with toxic debris and anerobic (unfriendly) bacteria, the lungs become congested with colds, flu, asthma, sinus congestion, pneumonia, chronic cough etc. The colon, digestive system and lungs are a complete respiratory system—they require oxygen and ozone to stay in good health and vitality.

The ancient masters taught that too much food in the G.I. tract blocks the lungs and respiratory system function from taking in pure prana, chi or ozone. Excess food in the gut, congests the blood, cells, tissues, and lungs/respiratory systems, and insulates the body cells against the natural contact of cosmic rays or natural radiation and ozone; it does this by corroding the poles of the cells. The telomeres at the end of your chromosomes become rusted or corroded, which accelerates the aging process. The cells require high level ozone/oxygen to function at a high level of health. Ozone is needed to slow you down from "rusting" or aging. At the cellular DNA/Telomere/Chromosome level, damage increases from too much food, especially junk food, smoking, alcohol, drugs, air pollution. Vital chi energy force slowly declines, and sickness, pain and decrepitude replace youthful vitality. When cells and telomeres corrode or rust, they fall to a low vibration rate, until all your cells die, and your form dissolves into the earth.

This is why fasting, whole body detox cleanses, and pure oxygen-ozone therapy, plus the FIR Sauna can help to cleanse your alimentary tract and respiratory/lung system of toxic debris, and release the insulating effect of undigested, rotting food in your G.I tract. The cells and telomeres can then be free of this cellular "rust" or corrosion—thus liberating and opening the life-enhancing air sacs in your lungs to keep you oxygenated and vital. We are first and foremost oxygen creatures; food and water are secondary. We were born with strong, robust lung capacity—a baby can yell all day and not get hoarse. Baby's lungs are clean and pure—not yet polluted by junk food and bad air. Heavy acid-forming foods, like animal foods, creates the most rust and corrosion in cellular structures, and weakens the organs and blood. Internal acidity lowers oxygen to your cells, and causes inflammation and pressure on all the internal organs, which causes chronic diseases. The cells need high level ozone and oxygen to keep the body buoyant, clear and healthy. Oxygen and breath are a spiritual function of existence. The Spirit of Life breathes through you to keep you enlivened and full of Life, Chi Force or Spiritual Force. We are not separate from Source Creation, nor can we ever be. We come from Creation and we never leave Creative Source or the God Force.

Having a clean body and colon, with oxygen/ozone flooding your cells, and with your lungs open, permits the body to make better use of the cosmic minerals and nitrogen, and returns you to a high state of health—your cells and telomeres can thus be filled with oxygen/ozone, and vibrate at high levels, like they were meant to, before the decline into modern junk food, ill-health and disease. Your health depends upon what you eat; what you eat determines the condition of your blood cells, which come from food. Your blood cells determine the condition of your body cells, tissues and organs; and the condition of all these factors depends ultimately upon the Breath of life—how you breathe and the quality of air you breathe-in on a daily basis. If all your cells are plugged-up and corroded, how can you expect to get inspiration, or "in-spir-ation," or "in-spiri-tualization" into your body? Were In-spir-ed when we perform re-spir-ation (deep breathing). Respiration is a spiritual process. All of life is a process of oxygenation, re-spir-ation, in-spir-ation on a biological and spiritual level, simultaneously. Your body is being "breathed" or in-spir-ed by the Universal One Spirit. No being or plant or animal on earth is exempt from being spiritualized, respirated and inspired by the spiritual force of the Universe. It is a natural process of spiritual life on earth.

We can't all live in the mountains, forest or seaside, where ozone is in abundance, but we can bring the ozone/oxygen to our home, with a fairly new device, the OxyOz Ozone Generator. This convenient, portable machine has several uses. It ozonates the air in your home. You can charge your water, tea, drinks, soups, smoothies with ozone. Ozonate your tub or juccuzi water, and you'll be charged with pure ozone while bathing. This is a "must have" device for your home or office, in this technical age of total pollution. We are bombarded with pollution everywhere now. You can make your home an ozone haven-zone. The OxyOz Ozone Generator, in combination with the FIR Sauna can help you lose weight by getting pure ozone/oxygen and FIR energy into your cells, tissues and lungs, thus detoxifying your colon, blood, liver and lungs in the process. You may find that you require and crave less food by breathing-in pure ozone into your system. The less toxins you have in your body, the easier it is to lose the pounds, and maintain a healthy weight, without overeating, or craving sweets. Turn on the OxyOz Generator, then sit in the FIR Sauna for 30 minutes—you'll get an accelerated energy, healing and detoxification boost beyond the ordinary. Order your OxyOz Ozone Generator. (Under $500). www.momentum98.com, (Phil Wilson) 800-533-4372. **Mention you read it here, and receive a discount.** If you're looking for superior health, detox, weight-loss, energy, call this number today! (See picture of OxyOz Ozone Machine next page).

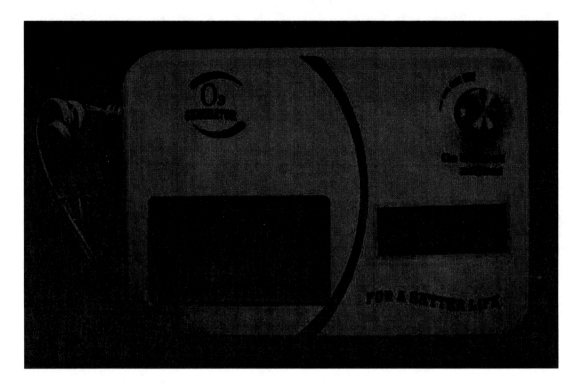

The first comprehensive Ozone Oxygen Mini-Spa System For Air, Water, Shower, and Bath

Specifications:
Model Name: OZX-300AT
Max. Ozone Output: 200mg/hr. without connection to TETRA WHISPER AIR PUMP. Ozone output: adjustable. Internal Air Pump output: 1-2L/min. Wattage: 10W. Timer: 60 min. (5 min. interval) and constant ON function. Pump Pressure: 17 Kpa. Ozone Generating Method: Corona Discharge (Ozone Tube). Gas Resource: Ambient Air. Air inlet Dim: 6.5mm. Outlet: Dim: 6.5mm. Power Source: AAC110-120V or AC220-240V. Body Size: 215mm x 60mm. Net Weight: 800g. Power Cable: 1-1.5mm in length. Accessories Included: 2 sets of hose diffuser

Application and Functions
- Purifying Drinking Water: Ozone can be pumped into a glass or bottle. As activated oxygen is created, it disinfects, enriches, and enhances the quality of water. After ozonating, let the ozone saturate the water for about 5-10 min, and break down to a more palatable water rich with ozone/oxygen. Great for tea, coffee, soups, and cooking. The taste is far better!
- Purifying fruits, vegetables, and meats, which are susceptible to agricultural and chemical residue. Simply put them in a container full of water, and diffuse the ozone into the water. Toxins with be significantly neutralized.
- Put bubbler into your bath, and attach the special Shower Head Filer to your shower. 1 year warranty. (Air pump not shown, but included in complete package).

Index

Abdomen, 59
Accommodation, 7
Accommodative Yoga exercise, 32, 33
Aceyl-L-Carnitine, 144
Acupressure-vision, 21, 22
Acupuncture, 122
Adrenal lands and sugar, 73
Adrenals and Kapha type, 81
Aerobics, 156
Air body type, 86
Aivanhov, Mikhael, 59, 60
Alcohol and Liver, 71
Almond oil, 77
Alpha Lipoic Acid, 133, 140-143
Alternate gaze, 113
AMD, 153
American Indians, 112
Amino acids and soy, 77
Aminoguanidine, 144
Amla, 141
Anger and Liver, 90, 106
Animal foods, 24, 88, 91, 138
Antioxidants, 154
Apt, Dr. William, 18
Arching Eyebrows, 103
Art of reading, 126
Ascorbates, 156
Aspartame, 138, 147
Assimilation, 67
Astigmatism, 23
Avacado oil, 77
Ayurveda, 60, 73, 79, 127, 128

Back exercise, 52, 53
Back to Eden, 112
Balding, 75
Barberry herb, 78
Barefoot walking, 123
Barley malt, 72
Bates, Dr William H., 7, 10, 25, 44, 48, 49, 97, 99, 100, 111, 126, 129
B-complex, 142, 158

Beans, 84
Belly Massage, 59
Beta carotene, 158
Beverages, 84, 91
Bilberry, 145
Bilberry, 71, 78, 133
Bioflavonoids, 144, 146
Black background, 47
Black Globe Palming, 47, 48
Black period eye gazing, 100, 131
Black velvet, 46, 48
Blindness, 156
Blurry vision, 138
Brain, 136
Blackness, 46, 47, 97
Bladder, 81
Blinking eyes, 116
Bloating, 81
Blockage, 97
Bloodstream pure, 111, 112
Blueberries and vision, 71
Bragg's Liquid Aminos, 77
Brain, 59
Breathe, 46
Breathing exercise, 108, 115
Brough, Beverly, 121
Buckwheat, 71

Calcium, 138
Calcium, 72
Canola oil, 72, 74, 75, 76
Carboh Yarates, 92
Carnosine, 139, 151, 158
Carotene, 153, 156
Carotenoids, 144
Carroll, Dr. Alexis, 129
Carrots, 70
Cataracts, 18, 133, 135-138, 145, 146, 148, 152, 153, 155
Cayce, Edgar, 70
Celtic salt, 73
Centering movement, 56, 103
Central energy, 60, 67
Central fixation, 24

Chee Soo, Professor, 110
Chewing food, 68, 69
Chi Kung and vision, 19
Chi Kung, 52, 64, 98
Chinese Medicine, 60, 122
Chrysanthemum, 71
Cigarettes and health, 71
Ciliary eye muscles, 7
Clear out toxins, 129
Close vision chart 2, 38
Close vision exercise, 30, 32, 33, 35, 36, 37, 38, 42, 100, 124
Close work, 104, 113, 114
Coconut oil, 78
Colds and flu, 80
Condiments, 84, 91
Constipation, 73
Contacts, 11
Cooked food, 69
CoQ10, 145
Corbett, Margaret, 95, 97
Corn oil, 77
Cortical Cataracts, 138
Cottage cheese, 83
Cotton seed oil, 77
Cousens, Dr., Gabriel, MD, 157
C-reactive proteins, 137
Cryptoxanthins & cataracts, 133
Culture of Death, 157
Cyanide and Soy, 76
Cysteine, 139

Daily eye training program, 51
Dairy, 83, 91, 139
Dandelion, 71
Dan Tein, 59
Dao-Yin eye massage, 22, 57, 58, 59, 61
Day dreamer, 111
Degeneration, 151
Depression, 62
Devi Payal, Swami, 127
Devitalized foods, 65
Diabetes, 73, 74, 136, 137, 149, 157
Diabetic Retinopathy, 154

Diapter, 11
Diarrhea, 62
Diet and health, 117
Digestion, 67, 68, 75
Disease process, 68
Disease, 72
Distance seeing 13, 14, 17, 100, 104, 112
Distant vision exercises, 30, 32, 33, 35, 40, 42, 43, 124, 125
DNA, 147
Do.In, 60, 61, 64, 117
Dry itchy eyes, 80, 86
Dynanmic relaxation technique, 98

Eating habits, 67, 114
Edema and water, 81
Edging eye technique, 132
Edging, 25
Egyptian Black Dot Technique, 29
Egyptian letter gazing, 30, 31
Eucalyptus and vision, 20
Exercise, 85, 89, 92, 101, 149
Exhaling Bull eye technique, 115
Eye anatomy, 9
Eye ball shape, 120
Eye beauty treatment, 121
Eye chart routine, 132
Eye diagnosis, 10
Eye diagnosis, 117
Eye diagram, 9
Eye exercise and moderation, 104, 105
Eye glasses, 10, 11
Eye gymnastics, 120, 121
Eye habits, 13
Eye healing massage, 58, 59
Eye improvement techniques, 95
Eye lid massage, 115

Eye muscle balance exercise, 30, 31
Eye muscle exercise, 128 161
Eye muscles weak, 14, 15
Eye muscles, 7, 113, 115, 120
Eye power gaze, 119
Eye pupil exercise, 124
Eye relaxing, 14
Eye routine—short and long, 101
Eye strain, 13, 16, 113
Eyebright herb, 71
Eyebrows, 103
Eyes and brain, 10
Eyes and sight, 10, 99
Eyes, and blood and nerves, 14; and close work, 15; and cramping, 15; and eating, 15; and oxygen, 15, 16; and distant gazing, 15, 16; and illness, 16; and rest, 16; and immune system, 16; and
poor lighting, 16; and reading, 17; and palming, 19; and massage, 22; and eyebrow stroking, 23; and squeezing, 24; and tear glands, 24, and naturopathic massage, 24; and exercises, 27, 28, 32, 33; and eye whipping, 36, 37; and tromboning, 37; and close point exercise, 37; and chart, 37;
Eyesight and food, 64, 65, 79, 82, 83, 84, 85, 87, 88, 89, 90, 91, 92,
Eyesight training outline, 129
Eyesight training schedule, 50
Eye-Xerciser, 92

Farsightedness, 10, 14, 23, 29, 31, 32

Fast food, 68
Fatigue, 105
Fats and liver, 71, 74, 85, 88, 92, 103
Fatty liver, 156
Fiber foods, 148
Fish, 69
Five element system 74, 79
Flax seed oil, 78
Flexibility, 98
Focusing eye exercise, 37, 113, 115, 131
Foods for health, 69
Foot slapping, 61, 62, 63, 64
Free Radicals, 137, 139, 142, 146
Fruits, 71, 73, 82, 103, 88, 90

Gall bladder and vision, 66, 78
Gall stones, 74
Gastro-intestinal tract, 77
Gazing eyes, 124
Ghee, 78
Ginko, 144, 145
Glaucoma, 135-138, 148, 151, 154, 155
Glutathione, 139-142, 146, 147, 153, 156, 158
Glycation, 136, 139, 147, 148, 151, 154
Glycemic foods, 154
Gowman, Kaye, 102
Grains, 83, 91, 153
Grapes, 90
Green color and eye health, 47
Green foods, 137, 145, 156
Green vegetables and vision, 47
Gretsky, Wayne, 43
Gut, 67

Hara massage, 60, 62, 63
Harvard Medical School, 152
Hauser, Gaylord, 94
Head lift technique, 25
Healing eye sound, 24
Health, 66
Healthy eye, 8

Heart, 64
Heat, 92
Helmholtz, Dr., 7
Herbal teas, 84, 88, 89, 91
Herbal wines, 89
Herbs, 74, 91
High blood pressure, 73, 108
Himalyan salt, 73
Honey, 72, 73
Hormones, 73
Hunger, 66, 67, 68
Hydrochloric acid, 147
Hydrogen peroxide, 146, 152
Hydrogenated oils, 74
Hyperbaric Oxygen, 156
Hypocrites, 65
Hypoglycemia, 64

Immune system and health, 67, 76, 77
Indigestion, 67, 87
Inflamed red eyes, 80, 89, 90
Inflammation, 71, 136
Inositol, 144
Insulin, 73
Iris, 8
Ironing face, 23
Irradiation, 75
Itchy eyes, 85

Jade hop exercise, 55
Jensen, Dr. Bernard, 123
Jordan, Michael, 43
Junk foods, 72

Kapha and fruit, 83
Kapha dosha type, 80, 81, 82, 83, 122, 153
Kapha health therapies, 84
Kelp, 73
Kidney exercise, 52, 53, 63
Kidney massage, 21
Kidneys and eyes, 117
Kidneys and water type, 81
Kloss, Jethro, 112

Laser surgery, 136
Lazy eight neck exercise, 28

Lear oil, 76
Legumes, 84
Lemon juice eye bath, 18
Lemon, 78
Let go and see, 45, 49, 107, 108
Licorice herb, 71
Liquids, vision and health, 82, 121
Liu, Da, Taoist Master, 118
Liver and eye herbs, 71, 78, 123
Liver and eyes, 10, 14, 66, 110, 117, 118, 122, 123
Liver cleansing foods, 123
Liver Massage, 21
Liver, vision and soy, 76
Long swing exercise, 95, 97, 98, 99
Lorenzo's oil, 76
Low Insulin Index, 157
Lust, Dr. Benedict, MD, 111
Lutein and vision, 133
Lutein, 153, 158
Lychii Gogi berries, 71
Lycopene, 153

Macrobiotic liver diagnosis, 122
Macula, 25
Macular degeneration, 135, 137, 138, 151-153
Magnesium, 145
Man the Unknown, 129
Manganese, 158
Maple syrup, 72
Margarine, 74
Massage belly, 59
Massage feet and vision, 89
Meat, health and vision, 103
Meditation and vision, 89, 92, 108
Medium length eye routine, 101, 102
Melatonin, 143
Mental clam and vision, 49
Microscopic type print, 6
Migraine headaches, 127

Milk thistle, 78
Minerals, 73, 84, 88, 92
Moderation, 81
Mucous, 80
Mules and vision, 96
Muscles, 98, 162
Mustard gas and canola oil, 76
Mustard oil, 89
Myopia myth, the, 126
Myopia, 17, 26
Myopics and age, 24, 103

N-Acetyl-L-Carnosine, 139, 140, 143, 156
Nails and health, 71
Nasal massage, 20
Nasal wash, 127, 128
National Academy of Science, 156
Natural eye exercises, 124
Naturopathic cure, 120
Naturopathic eye massage, 24
Nearsightedness, 10, 14, 17, 23, 40, 71, 72
Neck exercise and vision, 22, 25, 59
Nourish eyes, 129, 130
Now moment, 107
Nuclear Cataracts, 138
Nutritional body types, 79
Nutritional secrets, 65
Nuts, 69, 75, 84, 88

Oatmeal, 71
Obesity and fats, 74
Obesity and Kapha water type, 81
Oil enema, 89
Oils, 71, 74, 75, 84, 87, 88, 92, 103
Olive oil, 76, 78
Oregon Grape root and liver, 78
Original nature, 66
Otsuka, Dr. Jin, 72
Outdoor dwellers, 18, 19
Overeating, 66, 121
Oxidative damage, 155
Oxygen, 157

Pack, Johnny, 19
Palm eye massage, 23, 45, 46, 47, 48
Palming, 19, 22, 34, 45, 95, 97, 99
Pancreas, 72
Parsley and vision, 71
Peanut butter, 77
Peanut oil, 77
Peanuts, 77
Perfect Eyesight, 101, 102
Peripheral vision, 8, 124
Peterson, Stephanie, 102, 103
Photo-phobia, 96
Phyto-hema-glutinin, 75, 76
Pinhole Glasses 174-175
Pitta dosha type, 80, 89, 91, 153
Pitta lotions, 92
Pitta/Vata body type, 86, 90
Pituitary gland, 108
Plaque, 75
Poor eyesight, 67
Positive lens glasses, 125, 126
Positive thinking, 106, 107
Posture and reading, 16
Posture and vision, 52
Potassium, 145
Potassium, 73
Potato juice eye bath, 82
Progressive eye training, 50
Protein molecule, 75
Protein, 85, 88, 92
Ptyalin enzyme, 68
Pulse, 90
Pungent, 90, 91
Pupil, eye, 8, 9, 96
Purgation therapy, 92

Qigong exercise, 61
Quercetin, 144

Rag doll limp exercise, 98
Rape seed oil, 76
Raspberry, 71
Raw food, 90, 116
Reaching for heaven, 53, 54

Reading and eyes, 16, 114
Reams, Dr. Carry, 75
Red eyes, 110
Red eyes, 89, 90, 122
Reduce mental strain, 49
Rehm, Donald, S, 126
Relax brain and mind, 49
Relax eye muscles, 49
Relaxation, 46, 47, 48
Relaxed, 97, 98, 99, 103
Rest the eyes, 49
Rest, 81, 105
Riboflavin, 139, 142
Rice bran oil, 143
Rocine, Victor, 78
Rockerfeller Medical Institute, 129
Rofidel, Jean, 10, 60, 61, 117
Rose hips, 141
Ross and Rehner, Drs., 15, 111, 113, 115
Rub massage, 58

SAD Diet, 148, 155
Safflower oil, 77
Saliva, 68
Salt, 73
Sasaki, Dr., Natural Eye Doctor, 17
Scalp rubbing, 23
School and vision, 31
Seasonings, 88
Seeds, 69, 70, 71, 75, 84, 88, 91
Selenium and cataracts, 133
Selenium, 142, 158
Sentimental diseases, 62
Sesame oil drops, 121
Sesame oil, 78
Shaftsbury, Edmond, 24, 112
Sharp appetite, 90
Sharp focusing, 97
Sharp vision tracking exercise, 24
Short eye routine, 101, 102
Sight Without Glasses, 114
Sinus problems and vision, 20
Sinus problems, 103
Sit down palming

technique, 47
Sleep and eyes, 105
Snellen eye chart, 34
Snellen Eye Test, 6
Soaked seeds and nuts, 143
Sodium, 146
Solar plexus, 59, 60, 62
Sore eyes, 27
Sour taste, 87
Soy and animals, 77
Soy oil, 72, 74
Soy protein, 77
Soybeans, 74, 75, 76, 77, 118
Spices, 84, 88, 90, 92
Spine straitening movement, 53
Spirulina plankton, 92
Squash, 156i
Squinting, 103
Staring, 99
Steady eye, 119
Stomach massage, 21
Straining eyes, 10, 17
Strengthen eyes, 129, 130
Stress and eye health, 104
Stressed out, 68
Stretch your vision, 40, 41
Success formula, 106
Sucralose, 147
Sufi bear walk, 55, 56
Sufi eye exercise, 108
Sugar Blues, 72
Sugar, 103, 136, 154
Sun Sensitivity, 149
Sunflower oil, 78
Sunflower seeds, 19
Sunflower seeds, 70
Sunglasses and vision, 19, 96
Sunlight and vitamin D, 6, 8, 96
Sunning eyes, 95, 96, 99
Sunshine vitamin, 70
Sunshine, 18
Supplement Recommendations, 149
Supplements, 84, 88, 92
Sweet taste, 87, 89
Sweeteners, 88, 91
Sweets and vision, 10, 83
Swollen eyes, 118, 122

Tai Chi Rocker eye exercise, 33, 34, 36
Taoist eye exercise, 128
Taoist eye palming, 45
Taste buds, 67
Taurine, amino acid, 133,
139, 141
Teeth, 72
Telescopic vision, 6
Tension, 45, 97
Testimonials, 102
Thankfulness, 106, 107
The Tree of Life Rejuvenation Center, 157
Thin white line, 127
Thinking positive, 105
Thinking, 62
Thirst, true, 66
Three power centers, 59
Thyroid gland, 108, 118
Tibetan Peripheral Vision Technique, 43, 44
Tibetan Rejuvenation Rite, 53
Tilney, Dr. Frederick, 105
Tocopherol, 156
Tofu, soy, 77, 118

Tolmich, Mrs., 95
Tongue coating, 67
Toxic blood, 74
Toxic foods, 71
Tracking eye exercise, 24, 25
Tracking, 124, 131, 132
Trans fats, 155
Tromboning eye exercise, 37
True hunger, 67
Tumors, 71

Vata characteristics, 86
Vata dosha body type, 80, 85, 86, 153
Vata eye diagnosis, 122
Vata foods, 86, 87, 88
Vata/Kapha body type, 86
Vegetable detox, 78
Vegetables, 71, 90, 137, 157
Vegetarian protein powder, 87
Vegetarians, 75, 83
Verma, Dr., Vinod, 71
Vision defects, 75
Vision healing, 57, 151

Vision problems, 83
Vision wisdom, 110
Vision, 20-20, 12, 107
Vitamin B-12, 19
Vitamin B-2, 72
Vitamin D, 70
Vitamins A, C, E, eyes, 133, 139-142, 144, 146, 147, 149, 155, 158
Vitamins, 84, 92
Vogel, Dr., 16

Walking, 156, 157
Water and eyes, 10, 64, 85, 86, 116, 117
Water and kapha type, 81, 82, 85, 86
Water drinking, 81
Water reducing foods, 83
Watery eyes, 80, 121
Weak vision, 18, 70, 74
Weak voice, 86
Weightlifting, 98
Wheat germ oil, 142
Whipping eye exercise, 36, 37
White flour products, 72, 73
White flour, 136

Who needs glasses, 121
Whole foods, 69, 74

Yan Shou Shu, 112
Yang eye candle gazing, 20
Yellow eyes, 110
Yellow spot, 9
Yoga accommodation eye exercise 32, 33
Yoga breathing, 85, 89, 98
Yoga eye palming, 45
Yoga fetal palming technique, 46
Yoga nasal massage, 20
Yoga sun gazing, 19
Yoga, 89, 103, 156
Yoga-Ratnakara, 128

Zeaxanthin, 145, 156, 158
Zen mind, 107
Zen-Taoist Master Hyunoong Sunin, 61, 62
Zinc, 156, 158

About the Authors

Robert Zuraw, (1941-2006), studied with Helen Tulmich, an instructor in the Dr. Bates-Corbett school of visual education. from 1961-63. He also studied with Dr. Sasaki, a Natural Eye Doctor, from Ann Arbor, Michigan. From 1964 to 1966 he was a Sergeant Nurse in the Army in Viet Nam for thirteen months in Siagon. He assisted surgeons in major operations with medical instruments and emergency causality readiness. He graduated with honors from the Career Academy School of Famous Broadcasting for two years 1968-69. He was the President of the Michigan Vegetarian Society from 1967 to 1988. In 1985 he studied with Dr. Shen Wong in the Art of Chinese Flying Crane Chi Kung Yoga Meditation. In 1987, he became a Certified Instructor in the Tien Tao Chi Kung System from the Chinese National Chi Kung Institute, a one year course in Esoteric Chi Kung Exercises and Meditation. In 1990, Robert studied with Zen-Taoist Master Venerable Hyunoong Seunim, a Buddhist monk from the mountains of Korea and Tibet. From Master Hyunoong Seunim, he learned the Five Element Body Typing System, Taoist Nutritional and Herbal Medicine, Taoist breathing exercises, which helped him overcome a severe energy blockage imbalance. He learned the Taoist Sun-Do Meditation and Taoist Yoga Techniques, Dao-Yin Self-Massage and Body Typing Energy Analysis. Robert is the **Originator of the Zuraw Eyesight Improvement Course**. He was a Nutritionist-Herbalist-Wholistic Health Consultant, and a noted Palmist and Character Reader. He improved his vision from advanced progressive myopia (20-600 vision), which is legally termed blind without glasses (in the mid-1960) to better than 20-20 vision, before his untimely passing on December 14, 2006.

Robert Lewanski, aka R.T. Lewis, studied the Natural Hygienic System of Health, Diet, Fasting in 1971-72 under the direct supervision of Dr. Herbert M. Shelton and Dr. Virginia Vetrano, at Dr. Shelton's Health School in San Antonio, Texas. In 1973 he was Certified in Foot Reflexology by Dr. William Kenner, Dearborn, MI. Certified in Chinese Medical Massage by Dr. Shen Wang in 1988. Director of Health Force Center, Royal Oak, MI. Studied and practices Do-In (Dao-Inn) Self-Healing Massage, Acupressure, Swedish Massage, Cranial-Facial Massage, Shiatsu Oriental Massage for 20 years. In 1975-76, studied and graduated with high honors from Career Academy, School of Famous TV and Radio Broadcasters, Washington, D.C. President of the Detroit Chapter of the National Health Federation, 1977-79. In 1985, studied Flying Crane Chi Kung Yoga with Dr. Shen Wang. Certified Ayurvedic Counselor in Nutrition and Health from the Ayurvedic Institute, Albequerque, New Mexico, Dr. Vasant Lad, Director, Dr. Robert Svoboda, Chief Instructor. Studied Sun-Do Meditation, Chinese Five Element Nutritional Body Typing and Taoist Chi Kung Yoga from Master Hyunoong Suinum from Korea. He is a Tai Yoga Chi Kung Massage Therapist, Nutritional Chinese and Ayurvefdic Body Typing Consultant, noted Palmist, Character Reader and Personal Fitness Trainer from Troy, Michigan. He co-authored "Ancient Secrets of Health and Long Life," and "Health Force: The Art and Cultivation of Human Energy," with Robert Zuraw. He is also an organic food gardener.